Loose Threads

Loose Threads

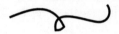

LORIE ANN GROVER

Margaret K. McElderry Books
NEW YORK   LONDON   TORONTO   SYDNEY   SINGAPORE

Margaret K. McElderry Books
An imprint of Simon & Schuster Children's Publishing Division
1230 Avenue of the Americas
New York, NY 10020

Book design by Russell Gordon
The text of this book is set in Aldine.
Printed in the United States of America
2 4 6 8 10 9 7 5 3
Library of Congress Cataloging-in-Publication Data
Grover, Lorie Ann.
Loose threads / by Lorie Ann Grover.
p. cm.
Summary: A series of poems describes how seventh grader Kay
Garber faces her grandmother's battle with breast cancer while
living with her mother and great-grandmother and dealing with
everyday junior high school concerns.
ISBN 0-689-84419-0
1. Breast—Cancer—Patients—Juvenile poetry. 2. Junior high
schools—Juvenile poetry. 3. Grandmothers—Juvenile poetry.
4. Cancer—Juvenile poetry. 5. Death—Juvenile poetry. 6. Children's
poetry, American. [I. Grandmothers—Poetry. 2. Breast—Cancer—
Poetry. 3. Cancer—Poetry. 4. Mothers and daughters—Poetry.
5. American poetry.] I. Title.
PS3557.R7428 L66 2002
811'.6—dc21
2001044724

Bible passages taken from American Standard Version, 1901 edition.

Dedicated to

MY GREAT-GRANDMOTHER, EULA MERCER,
1904–1986

MY GRANDMOTHER, MARGIE GARBER,
1921–1983

AND MY MOTHER, KARINE LEARY,
B. *1943*

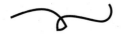

Special Thanks to

MY HUSBAND, DAVID GROVER;

MY PASTOR, TOM LYON;

AND MY EDITOR, EMMA DRYDEN

Loose Threads

M★A★S★H

Our living room
is cozied up with laughter.
Great Gran Eula smiles at the colonel
and sips her iced tea.
Grandma Margie snickers at Radar
over her knitting.
Mom laughs at Hot Lips
and doesn't finish paying the bills.
I laugh so hard at Hawkeye
my beanbag chair
squishes under me.
We finally stop laughing
during the commercial,
and Grandma Margie says,
"I found a lump
in my breast."

What They Know

"A lump?" I ask.
"On my left side."
"I'm sure it's nothing," says Gran Eula.
"Probably just fluid," says Mom.
"Certainly benign," says Gran Eula.
"We'll see," says Grandma Margie.
"I made a doctor's appointment."

All I'm thinking is,
I don't want to see or know
anything
about lumps
in Grandma Margie.

Breaking the Silence

"You didn't say
how school went today, Kay," Mom says.
"Fine," I mumble.
"Anything happen?" Grandma Margie asks.
"Not really," I say.
"What did you learn?" asks Gran Eula.

All that comes to mind is
Mr. Ball
spraying his air freshener
in English class,
trying to cover up his cigarette smoke
left over from break.
Tsssssssss,
till a cloud hovered
over us.
Smelled like
we were
in a flower field on fire.
"Most singular verb forms end in *s*,"
he chanted,
his big hair
cutting a passage through the room.

"Singular verb forms end in *s*,"
I finally answer.
"That they do," says Gran Eula.

Other Stuff

"Deb, Sheray, David, and I
are doing a science project
together," I add.
"Working as a team
is always fun," says Grandma Margie.
"Just don't let those three
leave you with all the work, sugarplum."
Gran Eula clinks her ice cubes
against her glass.
"Kay knows better than that," says Mom.
I squirm down in my beanbag chair,
remembering how I did do that
on last year's project.
I was the one who pinned
all those dead butterflies
to the cardboard
after I caught them
and killed them.
"No, we'll share the work," I say.
"I hope so." Gran Eula gives me
the eye.

What to Do

"Maybe we should discuss the lump," Mom says.
M★A★S★H comes back on.
None of us watch.
"Now, Karine," says Gran Eula,
"no need for that tonight."
"But—," says Mom.
"Karine."
Grandma Margie and I watch those two
go back and forth.
"But—,"
"Sh. Sh."
"Fine." Mom slaps the checkbook down.
"Fine my daughter will be," says Gran Eula.

Good Night

We missed the ending
of the show.
Grandma Margie clicks off the TV.
"Good night," says Gran Eula.
She carries her glass to the kitchen.
"Good night," says Mom,

leaving the pile of bills on the table.
"Good night," I tell Grandma Margie
even though it isn't one.
"Good night, Kay."
I look back.
Grandma Margie stays in her chair,
yarn between her fingers,
staring at her reflection
on the blank TV.

Bottles and Beauty

We brush our hair.
Natural pig bristles.
Brush our teeth.
Baking soda included.
Floss.
Waxed and minty.
Glop on cold cream.
Thick and white.
Rinse.
Tingly fresh.
Cake on mango masks.
Pink and gritty.

Smear on aloe lotion.
Smooth and soft.
Spray on flower scents.
Sweet and light.
All the stuff we do,
all the stuff we use,
to be healthy and beautiful
doesn't stop a lump
from growing,
I guess.

The Drawer

I open the bathroom drawer
to slip my brush in.
My fingers graze
their three brushes.
I pick up Grandma Margie's
and hold it close to my chest.
Her hair spray,
caught in the bristles,
smells clean.
Not like Gran Eula's,
whose smells chemically

and is tacky stiff.
One strand
of Grandma Margie's hair
tickles my cheek.
It matches my hair color
exactly.
I pull it from the brush
and pray,
"God, please make the lump
go away."
I lace the hair back into the bristles
and set the brush down gently
next to the others.
"Please, God."
I shut the drawer.
"Make it go away."

The Phone

I get the phone
and take it
to my bedroom.
I want to call Deb.

And tell her what?
My grandma has a lump?
How gross is that?
She'd say, "Where?"
And I'd have to say, "In her breast."
Or could I say "chest"?
Is that too lame?
Then she'd be thinking
about my grandma's breasts.
Then maybe mine next.
And what is that about?
Because there's no lump in mine.
That's for sure.
So forget it.
I put the phone back in the kitchen.
For-get-it.

2:00 A.M.

Grandma Margie stands at my door
in her robe and curlers,
looking at me in bed.
I fake sleep

till she walks away,
because I don't know what to say.
I can only pray.

We've Lost

Great-Grandfather
before I was born,
Grandpa
when I was five,
and Dad left
when I was six.
We can't
lose Grandma Margie
next.

Comfort

It is so cold
with the air-conditioning
turned down to sixty degrees.
Gran Eula always says,
"It's the only way

to sleep comfortably."
I slip outside onto the front porch.
The night air
is sweet and thick from mango blossoms.
The heat burrows through my skin
until I lean against our cool concrete house.
A warm breeze rustles the palm fronds,
then slips by my cheek
like a deep sigh.
And I am finally
able to sigh back.
Inside
I climb under my covers.
The warm air
still clings to my skin.
I fall asleep
smelling
mangoes.

Fine

I shift my backpack
so it stops
cutting
into my shoulder.
I'm walking out the door
into the steamy sunshine,
and Mom asks,
"You all right, hon?"
I don't answer.
"Kay?"
"Yeah," I say,
not meaning it.
"I'm fine."
For some dumb reason
I have to blink fast
to get rid of some stupid tears.
I've never been good at
saying how I feel
or showing I need anyone,
least of all Mom.
She's so perfect
she never even cries.
"I'm totally fine."

I swallow
and walk away
like I'm supposed to.

It Seems Like

Mom was the same
back when Dad was around.
Maybe she was too perfect
for him
to stay
around
us.

One Thing I Remember

Whenever Dad came home from work,
Mom always said,
"Put your shoes on the rack."
And he never did.
So I would
before she
could tell him again.

Mom needs everything around her
just right.
Even a row of shoes.
So,
Dad's shoes were right there
on the shelf
the day
he took them
and left.
Right where Mom told him
to put them.
Right where I put them.
Right there for him
to find them
and walk away
from her row
of shoes.

Work

A pebble skitters
off my shoe.
I shrug my backpack higher.

Gran Eula always says,
"Going to school
is your work for now, sugarplum."
It sure is work.
It's so big to her
because she only got
to the sixth grade.

She likes to remind me,
"We each have to contribute."
But what does my schooling
add to our home?
No one ever tells me that.

I yank a cherry from the neighbor's hedge
and chew off the sour flesh.
Thp.
The white seed bounces,
then sticks to the sidewalk.

I don't love school
like Mom loves accounting.
She loves working from home
on her computer.

And Grandma Margie loved working
as a seamstress
until she retired.

Once Gran Eula married,
she never worked
outside her home again.
"Always thought I had enough
good hard work to do in it."
That makes Mom humph
and Grandma Margie say, "Now, now."

With Mom's paycheck,
Grandma Margie's retirement money,
and us living in Gran Eula's house,
we make our bills.

My schoolwork
isn't near as fun
as the stuff they get to do.
I don't know what I'll work at
when I grow up,
but I want to make
a lot of money
so I can maybe
live alone.

Sometimes
that
sounds
nice.

Mosquitoes

"Come on, bus."
The younger kids and I
are sweating
and smacking
mosquitoes.
"Ouch!"
The horde moves in a gray cloud
from one of us
to the next.
None of us can stand still,
or we'll be covered.
"Man!"
Slap, smack, slap.
"Come already," a little kid whines.
"Hurry," I say.
We beg the bus to come
around the corner

before there's nothing
of us left
to pick up.

The Bus

Rock,
bump,
creak,
hisssss.
The cool bus window
feels good
against my hot forehead.
I only move to scratch
my mosquito bites.
Everyone's pretty quiet
so early in the morning.
"Hi, Kay," is all Deb and Sheray say
as they slip into their usual seat
behind me.
"Hey," I say back
without lifting my head.
David
sits in the back today.

Every morning I pray
that he'll sit next to me.
He's so cute.
But today
I'm thinking about Grandma Margie,
and I don't care
where he sits.
Hattie's the last to get on.
She takes her usual seat
behind the driver.
The seat that no one else
wants to sit in.
We rock,
bump,
creak,
hisssss,
scratch
all the way to school.

Bites

In homeroom,
Ms. Reynolds
calls attendance.
I poke my fingernail
into the biggest mosquito bite
on my arm.
First one way,
then another.
Crisscross
through the lump.
I turn it
into a star.
But the poison oozes up again.
The star disappears,
and I'm only left with
a redder lump
that itches worse.

Poison

Is there
poison like this
in Grandma Margie's lump?
Poison that looks like it goes away
when it's crisscrossed
but comes back
before you know it?
I lick my thumb
and cover my mosquito lump.
My spit cools it off.
I'm not going to scratch it
anymore.

"Kay Garber," calls Ms. Reynolds.
"Here," I answer,
and scratch the lump
without thinking.

Science

Ms. Certel
is always on a diet.
A water diet this time.
Laughing,
she runs to the bathroom
because of eight, nine, ten glasses of water.

We go nuts when she leaves,
throwing paper,
boys belching,
girls shrieking.
Even I
can forget about Grandma Margie
for a minute
and laugh as loud
as anyone
until Ms. Certel comes back.
"Do I need to remind you
you are now in junior high?
Please, class."
But she smiles
when she turns
to the board.

We love
Ms. Certel
and her water diet.

The Project

We're divided into project groups.
"So, what do you want to do?" David asks.
I shrug and look away
from his blue eyes.
Real cool,
but my face is warm.
My hands leave sweat marks
on our black tabletop.
I quickly slide my folder
over the wet spots.
"The butterfly project
was great last year," says Deb.
She flips her long hair
behind her shoulder.
Sheray and David say, "Yeah."
No one tells him
how that was my, Sheray, and Deb's project.
Or that I did everything.

"Let's think of something
really good," says Sheray.
She slides a bead
up and down one of her braids.
"I know," says David.
"How 'bout
we trace around each other?
We can do life-size drawings
of the different stuff inside us."
"That sounds like a lot of drawing," I say.
"No, we can do it!" Deb claps her hands.
"Do you mean like
the circulatory system?" asks Sheray.
"Yeah, and the muscles,
and the skeleton," David adds.
"And the organs," I whisper.
With lumps.
Can I tell them
about Grandma Margie?
David nudges me.
"You could act a little more excited," he says.
I smile.
I can still feel where his elbow poked me.
"Okay."
There's no way

I can tell them
with David here.
"Are we going to draw,
you know,
everything?" Deb giggles.
David grins. He has great teeth.
"Just the inside stuff!" he laughs.
"I'll do the circulation," says Sheray.
"I'll do the muscles," says David.
"I'll do the skeleton," says Deb.
The three of them stare at me.
"I'll do the organs," I say.
"All right!" David smiles.
Right at me.

Study Hall

I finish the fantasy novel
we were assigned to read
and smooth the curling cover.
If I had a potion,
or a crystal ball,
I'd fix everything.
I'd heal Grandma Margie

and maybe bring the men
from my family back.
A spitball flies past my nose.
I glance around
but don't have a clue
who spit it.
Everyone is reading.
I bet they wish
they had
a potion
or a crystal ball too.
But all we've got
are spitballs.

The Lunchroom

I dump out my pork rinds.
Now's the perfect time to tell
about Grandma Margie.
Deb and Sheray
are the only ones
at the table.
They are laughing

at the guys behind us
tossing Hattie's lunch bag around.
I eat a rind
super loaded with hot sauce.
My mouth is on fire.
I can't tell them anything.
I gulp my milk
even though
it tastes sour.

Real Stuff

School rolls on.
Class after class.
Teachers give assignments.
It's so fake
when real stuff is going on.
Like David dumping Sue Lyn.
Like Liz and Dwight both having mono.
Like Buff getting caught smoking pot
with Levena under the bleachers.
Real stuff
like kids in trouble,

and families growing lumps.
School rolls
over
us.

Routine

"The doctor says
I need to have a biopsy," says Grandma Margie.
"But I didn't even know
you went to the doctor," I say.
"I didn't want to worry you."
She spoons some mashed potatoes onto her plate.
"Grandma Margie . . ."
I try to keep my voice quiet.
"I want to know when stuff happens, okay?"
"Now, now, sugarplum," Gran Eula cuts in.
"That is that, and this is this.
She just told us about the biopsy."
"Yes, she did," says Mom.

I stab a lima bean.
"So, what is a biopsy?" I ask.
"It's when they use a little knife or needle

to remove tissue
to test it," says Grandma Margie.
I drop my fork.
The lima bean holds on,
but a piece of my chicken-fried steak
bounces onto the table.

"Nothing to worry about," says Gran Eula.
She dabs her forehead with her napkin.
"She'll be fine," says Mom.
She puts the meat
back onto my plate.
"It's routine," Grandma Margie says to me.
"Go ahead and finish eating."

Eat?
I can't even swallow
this one shriveled
lima bean.

Checking

I spit into the sink.
"What does 'test it' mean, Mom?"
She takes the hot washcloth
from her face.
"Oh, you know. Check the cells.
Make sure they're growing okay."
I rinse my toothbrush
and drop it in the hole
next to Grandma Margie's.
"Are they checking
for cancer?"
"Shh, Kay!"
Mom wrings out her cloth.
"Don't even mention that!"
I rip off
a piece of floss.
Biopsy
definitely means
checking
for cancer.

The Biopsy Appointment

They look away
from the red circle on the calendar.
Gran Eula vacuums by it.
Grandma Margie dusts around it.
Mom walks quickly past it.
But I get stuck in front of it.
That circle squeezes my chest
tight.

The Porch

I lean
against the house
and shuffle my homework.
Little kids play
boxball in the street.
Their shouts hang
in the thick air.
The sun shoots red streaks
across the sky,
and our orange porch tiles are still warm
from the hot day.

My sweaty footprints
evaporate.
I brush off a few no-see-ums.
Across the street
the house's glittery mica paint
sparkles brightly.
The lizards creep out
before I realize
I haven't done
a bit of homework.
Someone will be calling me inside
any minute for a report
on what I have done.
"Nothing" is the answer,
but only the lizards will know.
I zip through four pre-algebra problems
before I hear,
"Kay."
The lizards run.
The sun sets,
and I go in,
shutting the door
on the mosquitoes
who are just waking up
and ready to bite.

Everyone Knows

Gran Eula told her bridge club.
Grandma Margie told her prayer group.
Mom told her bowling league.
By now
it's gotten around church,
school,
and our neighborhood.
Everybody knows.
Nobody knows
I wasn't ready
for anyone else
to know.

Talking with Deb and Sheray

I take a deep breath
and turn around on the bus.
"So," I say.
"Yeah," they say.
"It's in her, um . . . ," I say.
"Yeah, we heard," they say.
"She's going to be—," I say.

"Okay," they say.
"Yeah," we say.

Before School

Deb, Sheray, and I
hang out in the school library.
It feels like we are popular and in
when we sit together.
No one notices us
in a bad way.
Plus,
we can look out the window
and see the really in kids,
the totally popular ones
like David,
standing around the front flagpole
until the bell rings.
We can see
who is talking to who,
whisper about who is liking who.
"I don't see David," I say.
"Hi." He touches my arm,
and I yelp.

He laughs.
"Hey, Kay. What's up?"
"Nothing."
He smiles at me,
then walks over to the magazine section.
I press my hands to my burning, hot face,
while Deb and Sheray giggle
into their books.

A Good Day

Aced the science test.
Finished my English essay
on the poet Anne Bradstreet.
Ran the mile in ten minutes.
It's a good day.
Maybe because it started with Deb and Sheray
not laughing or being grossed out
about Grandma Margie's lump.
That really
made the day
good.

After School

We decide to walk home.
Maybe because we are next to each other
and don't have to look at each other,
we can talk about breasts.
"My mom's was benign," says Deb.
"And my Granny Alma
just had fluid in her lump," says Sheray.
"That's great."
We step off the curb
and cross the street.
Are they thinking
of Mrs. Carter,
our second-grade teacher,
who died
from breast cancer?
If they are,
they aren't saying so.
Me, either.

The Roach Mobile

The Roach Mobile
is parked in our driveway.
"Bye," says Sheray.
"See you later," says Deb.
They hurry past,
trying not to look
at it.
Everyone probably needs the Roach Mobile.
But no one ever talks about it.
The giant plastic roach
antennae
dangle over the windshield.
The Roach Man
must be inside
with the chemical tank
on his back,
spraying stinky fumes
into every corner
and baseboard.
Grandma Margie
hates roaches.
I hate the Roach Mobile
sitting in the driveway,

telling everyone
we have roaches.
If those fumes kill roaches,
what do they do to people?
Do they make lumps grow?
There's no way Grandma Margie
will wait outside with me.
She watches the Roach Man
the whole time
to be sure he doesn't miss
a spot.
I climb up into the sea grape bush
and wait for the creepy guy to leave.
No one can see me
keeping an eye
on that giant plastic roach.

Rules in Junior High

"You are not allowed
to be going out,"
says Mom.
"To be dating,"
says Grandma Margie.

"To be courting,"
says Gran Eula.
Courting?
What's that?
All I said was
David has
a really nice smile.
And now
no one
is smiling.

Way Easier

It was so way easier
last year
in sixth grade.
Some girls
wore makeup.
Some girls
wore bras.
Some girls
were going out.
But some weren't.

Now if you don't
do all of that,
you'll be noticed.
This year
it feels like
any second
they could start noticing
me.
Then picking on me.
But so far
I'm still in,
at least with Deb and Sheray.
No one's made fun
of me
for not going out.
I don't hate it my family's so strict.
Except when I think
of how really cute
David is.

Memorizing

My Sunday School teacher,
Miss Martha Faye,

is so beautiful.
I memorize how
her blue eyeliner follows her eyelid,
where her green eye shadow
starts and stops,
and how her dark red lip liner
disappears into
her lighter red lipstick.
And then
I memorize my Bible verse.

Sunday Morning

We girls always claim the third pew
and save each other seats.
Deb doesn't go to church,
but Sheray does,
and today she saved me a spot
on the end.
I fidget.
Sometimes panty hose
are so uncomfortable.
Sheray is busy taking notes.
Her dad makes her do that.

"'Blessed are the dead
who die in the Lord,'" quotes our pastor.
I pull the hose off my shin
and it snaps back.

"'And he shall wipe away
every tear from their eyes;
and death shall be no more.'"

I bend over to scratch my ankle
and get a look at my family
across the aisle.
Gran Eula is nodding her head yes,
with her eyes closed.
Grandma Margie is smiling up at our pastor.
Mom is holding her Bible to her chest.
I forget my itch
and sit up straight.
I should pay better attention.
Shame holds me still
the rest of the hour.

Sunday Evening

"Another good day
of preaching," says Grandma Margie.
"I love evening service as much as morning."
"Me, too," says Mom.
She accelerates to pass an old truck.
Our headlights cut into the hot darkness.
Gran Eula tugs her sleeves from her armpits.
"Well, the service was nice,
but this humidity isn't.
My shields are soaked.
Open the windows."
She reaches up front
and punches off the air conditioner.
"At least we can get some air
moving through here."
In the rearview mirror
I see Mom roll her eyes.
But she still buzzes all the windows down.
"See?" says Gran Eula,
raising her voice over the wind.
"That is better," says Grandma Margie.

Scuttling

We turn onto Old Cutler Road,
by the bay.
Gran Eula's talk radio turns staticky.
"Oh, I forgot it's mating season," groans Mom.
Land crabs race across the street
to get inland.
Mom grips the steering wheel.
Gran Eula grips her pocketbook.
Grandma Margie grips the dashboard.
I grip my bottom lip between my teeth.
We are going thirty miles per hour,
and twelve-inch crabs are racing
across the road
every which way.
"Karine, look out!" Gran Eula hollers.
Mom swerves
right,
left, right, left,
right,
not caring for the crabs in love,
but caring for our tires.
None of us wants to put the spare on
in the dark

with these feisty crabs in heat
around our ankles.

CRUNCH

We don't breathe.
The tires hold.
"Would you take a gander
at that," says Gran Eula.
One crab is standing
smack in the middle of the road.
He lifts his claws
for a showdown with our headlights.
Mom drives straight ahead.
Our wheels
run on either side of him.
I look out the back window.
That one tough crab
is still in the middle of the road,
scuttling forward
to attack
the next car.

The Biopsy

They make me go to school.
The whole morning
I'm thinking, *Needle.*
I'm thinking, *Knife.*
I'm thinking, *Stitches.*
At lunch I call home from the school office.
"She's resting comfortably," says Gran Eula.
"Okay," I say. "Are you sure?"
"Yes," she says. "Here, talk to your mother."
"Is she okay, Mom?"
"Of course, hon.
Now, you get to class
and focus on your work."
"Okay. But would you tell Grandma Margie
I love her?"
"Yes, Kay. That's very nice."
"And I love you, too, Mom."
"Yes, honey, I know. Now, go to class."
We hang up.
A tiny part of my mind
notices
Mom didn't say

she loves me back.
But she did say
Grandma Margie's okay.

The Water Fountain

I stop by the fountain
and swallow medicine
for my cramps.
That should take away
the crunching pain.
I hardly noticed it earlier,
being so worried.
Does Grandma Margie
feel pain right now?
Have they given her medicine
to stop it?
I wipe the water off my chin
and hurry to the bathroom.
The medicine
feels like it's working
already.

Safer

Sue Lyn got her period in fifth grade.
No one could believe it.
The rest of us
got ours in sixth and now seventh.
Everyone
but Hattie.
Kids laugh at her
just because
she's flat.
None of them
think of
breast cancer
and how,
for right now,
Hattie's
safer than us.

Pre-algebra

"Two x plus four y."
We get the simple formula,
but Mr. Arnold
drones
on and on
about x and y,
and x and y,
and x and y,
and equations.

The class
passes notes
about Cindy and David,
and Cindy and David,
and Cindy and David
being the equation.

A Little Incision

"It will heal quickly," says Gran Eula.
"I'm sure," says Mom.
Grandma Margie nods.
When they turn away,
Grandma Margie grimaces.
But when she sees me looking,
she quick smiles.
I try to still my shiver
and smile back.
"Boy, it's cold in here," I say,
and rub my goose-bumpy arms.
"Do you want a blanket, Grandma Margie?"
"Please," she says.
I tuck a soft knit blanket
around her narrow shoulders
carefully.

Questions

I want to ask:
What's it feel like
to have part of a lump of you
cut out?

It's a part of you
that grew,
and now it's gone, right?
Do you miss it?
Can you tell it's gone?
Is it like a hangnail
you can't wait to cut off?
But a hangnail can't hurt you
like a lump.
Aren't you so relieved
it's mostly cut out?

But all I can ask is:
"Coffee, Grandma Margie?"

She's Up

She's careful with the spot.
Keeping her arm tucked close
over where her stitches must be.
But she's up,
doing the usual,
tidying and knitting.
Maybe this lump

isn't such a big deal.
But
I'm going
to keep
watching.

Waiting

Pretending we aren't waiting,
we act
through meals—
    Gran Eula makes her beans and corn bread,
through church—
    Mom teaches Sunday School to the
    second graders,
through mornings—
    Grandma Margie reads her Bible,
and evenings—
    we go for walks.
We act like we aren't waiting
for Grandma Margie's biopsy results.
But it's the only thing
we're waiting for.

Not that Bad

When Gran Eula
plays her classical records,
it's not that bad.
The music is gentle and soft
and makes me kind of sleepy.
When Grandma Margie
has her big-band TV show on,
it's not that bad.
The trumpets are loud
and talk back and forth
in bursts.
And when Mom turns the radio
to the classic rock station,
it's not that bad.
The beat is strong
even if the lyrics are stupid.
But nothing is better
than lying on my bed
with my headphones on,
listening to my own CDs.

Researching

"There's a ton of stuff inside us."
"Let me see." Deb pulls the book
across the library table.
Sheray's braids clink
as she pulls her chair close.
"There sure is," says Deb.
"It's going to take forever
to draw all those organs," I whine.
"Yeah." Sheray looks up.
She points out the window at David.
"But you get to work with him."
We grin.
"Maybe forever
isn't so bad."

What I See

I shouldn't peek
around the bathroom door,
but it's cracked open
just enough for me to see
Gran Eula

in her big bra and girdle
standing in front of the mirror
crying,
with the faucet gushing
so no one hears.
But I see
her tug those straps up,
first one side,
then the other,
snap her girdle at the waist,
splash her face,
and turn off the spigot.
That's all I see
because I'm too embarrassed
to watch anymore.
I tiptoe away
before she hears
me looking.

The First Knitting Lesson

"This is a good time to learn,"
Grandma Margie tells me.
"Okay." I focus on the two long needles
in her hand.
"You know,
I never could teach your mother."
I look up. "Really?"
"She's right handed, and I'm left."
"For once it's good to be a lefty," I say.
"It's great to be a lefty."
She casts on for me.
The yarn wraps onto one needle.
"So whose fault was it really
that Mom didn't learn?"
"Oh, both our faults, I guess."
I watch the yarn bunch down the metal.
"But it did seem like your mother
had eleven fingers sometimes."
I smile.
Eleven isn't perfect.

Mistakes

The hole is huge.
"Pull it out," says Grandma Margie.
"You dropped a few stitches."
I just sit there.
She takes the needles
and unravels
my hour of work
in five seconds.
The wiggled, bent yarn
is in a pile
on my toes.
"Now, start again from here."
She hands me the needles.
I slide one
against the other,
hook a stitch,
loop over,
slip it off one needle,
then the other.
The yarn knots.
"Don't yank it," says Grandma Margie.
It sticks to my moist fingers.
"Man," I mutter so I don't tear up.

"It's okay," she says,
looping the yarn over the needle for me.
"It's going to be okay."
I nod
and try to believe her.

Study Hall

I love knowing
who likes who,
and who's going out,
even if I just get
to pass the note
and I'm not going out
with anyone.
I fold the crinkled paper
up again
and pass it on to Christie.
At least
I'm cool enough
that they let me pass
the notes.

Why?

No one knows
why
we hate Hattie.
Maybe it's her wool skirts
and kneesocks.
Maybe it's because
she's the last to develop.
Maybe it's because
she makes A's.
Maybe it's because
if we hate her,
no one
will hate us.

Tracing

"Keep the noise down
while you work
on your projects, people," says Ms. Certel.
Each group
gets a little quieter.

I unroll the four huge sheets of paper
I got from the art room.
"I'll trace you," David says to Deb.
"Great." She lies down on a piece of paper.
"This is going to be
such a cool science project," says Sheray.
"Hm," I say. "I'll trace you, I guess."
"Okay," she says.
The whole time I'm going around Sheray
with a marker,
I'm looking over at Deb and David.
He's swept her long hair
to one side
to outline it.
She's giggling a lot,
and he's happy.
I should be happy too.
We are all working together.
I'm not doing the whole project alone.
I'm just not exactly
getting to work with
who I wanted.

Favorite Pastime

Grandma Margie and I
walk to the canal
with our poles
and white bread.
Flip, flap, flap.
Our flip-flops are gummy
on the hot asphalt.
We sit under the palm tree's
skinny shade
and squish bread
into perfect dough balls,
then hook them.

Slowly
we lower balls
into the water,
and the fish nibble
until the hook is empty.

We never really mean to catch one.
We only want to watch
them nibbling

and feel good
because
we are feeding them.

Making Chicken Pot Pie

Mom stops working early.
"I'm going to start dinner," she says.
"How about chicken pot pie?"
"Okay," I say.
Uh-oh.
Pie crust
is the one thing
that makes Mom
lose her cool.
She frowns
and huffs.
The crust rips and tears.
She has to roll
it out again.
It's getting tougher
every second,
and so is she.
She might even curse

for the first time
without spelling it.
"C-R-A-P," I heard her spell once.
She was steamed at the IRS.
Gran Eula, Grandma Margie, and I
go to our rooms
because if we
snicker once,
we might finally
hear the word
and end up wearing
the pie crust.

Click

Grandma Margie says to meet her later
at the diner.
She's going to the doctor's alone.
So Mom drives me and Gran Eula.
Click, click.
Click, click.
Mom glares at me in the rearview mirror.
"Would you stop that clicking?"
"But I'm not—," I start.

"I'm sorry, Karine. That was me."
Gran Eula closes her pocketbook. *Click.*
Mom looks straight ahead at the traffic.
Click.
Click, click.
Gran Eula
starts clicking
her pocketbook
again.

Telling

I swallow.
The soda burns.
Grandma Margie tears
the instant-coffee packet open
like she hasn't just said,
"I have cancer."

Clink, clink
goes her spoon
above the diner chatter.
Grandma Margie's coffee spins,
and she picks
at a loose thread

in her sweater.
It unravels.
"We'll have to fix it," says Gran Eula.

Sweetness

Gran Eula
is so harsh and strict.
Mom is such
a perfectionist.
What
are they about?
It's Grandma Margie who
is sweet.
Her pure sweetness
connects each of us
to the other.
Her plain sweetness
holds us together.

It's like my family
is the slice of key lime pie
Gran Eula's stopped eating.
She's the crust.
Mom is the sour, tangy lime filling.

I'm the lime circle slice
splat on top,
and Grandma Margie is the sugar.
The very sweetness that makes us
delicious.

Silently

God, I'm still asking you
to make it go away.
Not just the lump,
the cancer.
All the specks.
Please,
make them disappear
out of my Grandma Margie.
Every last molecule.
Please?

Fault

My fingers slide down
my sweating glass.
Is it my fault?
Because I didn't pray enough before?
I was thinking
so much about my stuff:
the science project,
Deb and Sheray,
homework,
and David.

"Didn't we pray hard enough?" I ask.
The three of them look at me.
I bite my lip.
I've said something
wrong
for sure.

"Sugarplum"—Gran Eula rubs her forehead—
"we don't control God with prayer."
"Absolutely right," says Mom.
"Hon, He's not like a vending machine in the sky
that when we pray,
out comes

whatever we want."
"Our part
is the prayer part," says Grandma Margie.
"Then we trust him
to do what's best." Gran Eula
dabs her napkin
on her lips.

"But how can the lump being cancer
be what's best?"
"We'll have to wait to see." Gran Eula
raises an eyebrow.

How can
cancer
ever
be for the best?

Choices

It sounds like she's reading
off the diner menu,
but this is a cancer menu,
and she can decide
what she wants.

"Radiation,
chemotherapy,
lumpectomy,
partial mastectomy,
or full," she says.
Nothing at all
sounds delicious
on this menu.

Looking out the Window

I wish
I could still ride a trike.
Three wheels
holding me up,
not having to think of balancing,
and no one telling me
what's really going on,
because I'm too young.
I wish
I still
rode a trike.

Can't

The bus groans.
I look straight ahead
when Deb and Sheray
get on.
They'll find out
cancer's
in Grandma Margie.
Everyone will talk
like last time,
until even my friends
hear.
I don't need to tell them.
I can't.

The Next Second

The last stop.
Hattie gets on
and sits up front.
I doodle the word
CANCER
on my history notes.

"Did you do the science . . ."
Deb lets go of the back of my seat.
Sheray peeks over.
"It's cancer!" one of them whispers.
I close my notebook.
It's funny how sometimes
you do something
a second ago
you didn't think
you ever could.

Limp

Deb hurries to catch up to me.
"I'm so sorry."
"Yeah."
Sheray matches my step.
"It'll be okay."
"Maybe."
The flag hangs limp
this morning.
"Deb," calls David.
My friends stop
to talk to the kids

by the flagpole.
I walk into the school
alone.

Preparation

Mom reads piles of books.
Books on cancer,
books on treatments,
whole books
about breasts.

Gran Eula interviews doctors.
"This one is good for bedside manner.
But this one is offering
experimental medicines for studies.
And this one offers holistic practices
and traditional medicines."

Grandma Margie and I go for walks
and talk about
my science project,
my friends,
and how we love the purple
in the sunset.

We talk about
everything
but cancer.
That's
important too.

Looking

"Did you ever notice
you have your Great Gran Eula's nose, Kay?"
"Yeah," I admit.
Grandma Margie leans close
to me on the front porch steps.
She looks like she's made
of all different gray colors
because the sun has set.
"Boy, the crickets are chirping
loud tonight," I say.
Who wants to look like their great-grandmother?
"Your noses are just alike," she insists.
"Hard," I laugh. "We are both hard-nosed."
"That's not what I meant."
She brushes my bangs back,
takes my face in her hand,

and turns my head
to look at my profile.
"I can see the similarity
so clearly in the moonlight."
Her fingers tremble
on my chin.
"But I have your eye shape,
and we have
the same color hair," I say.
She lets go.
"It's too dark to compare."
I hold her hand
until it stops trembling.
"There's a lot of me
that I got from you, Grandma Margie."
She leans her head on my shoulder.
And whispers, "Thank you."

Suspicious

Whenever Grandma Margie
has been out of the house,
and we come back home,
she checks all the closets

and under all the beds.
Every time
she has to make sure
no one has snuck in
and is waiting to get us
and steal our stuff.
We look away
till she's done.
We act like we don't notice her weirdness.
What makes her so afraid
she has to check
every time?
When she was little,
did someone hide under her bed,
then jump out and scare her?
Did someone rob her?
"Forget about under the bed!"
I want to yell.
The cancer has already
snuck in!
When you weren't looking,
this microscopic burglar
slipped into your very own body
to steal your life!
Be afraid of that, already!

The Cool Cloud

After school
I climb up into the sea grape bush
to read.
"Kay, come!" Mom calls.
I eat one of the last
powdery purple grapes left,
close up my book,
and jump down.
All the other kids run too.
"Hurry, Kay," Mom says.
Shhhhhhhh. The mosquito truck
is getting close.
Mom shuts the door
just in time.
We watch out the window
as the truck
moves down our street.
The white cloud
shhhhhhhhes out behind it.
The flashing red light
barely slices
the smoke.

The sound gets faint,
but the smoke hangs between the long roots
of the banyans,
which stretch from the treetops
down to the grass.
It weaves under the spiky palmetto leaves
and around the sea grape bush's leaves,
which look like big hands
trying to push it away.
Two kids whoop it up
and race after the truck.
My mom's breath catches.
"Don't you know about cancer?"
I want to ask them.
The boys run into the cool cloud
and disappear.
The mosquitoes are dead.

Mom and Me Love Bowling

Mom sips her soda
and jots down my split.
I slide onto the molded plastic seat
and watch her

prepare for a strike.
Little hip wiggle,
two tiny steps,
three big ones,
release,
and
strike.
Of course.
High five walking past me
to the bench.
My turn.
Gutter ball.
"You're doing fine, Kay," she lies.
"Concentrate, honey."
My ball bursts back up the ramp
and rolls to a stop.
I plug the holes
and hurl the ball
at the pins.
Thump,
thump.
It leaps a lane
and gutters again.

"That's better," says Mom.
And we bust up
laughing.

Time

What will Grandma Margie
finally decide
is the right thing to do
about the cancer?
"It's okay to take time
to sort everything out,"
Gran Eula says to her
during dessert.
Mom nods.
I smash my candied cherries
with my fork.
I hate their fake red sweetness.

Peach

My history teacher,
Mr. Hoeksema,
called me a peach today.
"Kay, you are a peach," he said
in front of everyone.
Just because I offered to lend my notes
to Hattie, who's missed some school.
Everyone knows
Mr. Hoeksema is cool.
He lifts weights in the gym
with the football team.
He's only twenty-four or something
and can totally relate to us.
So now
I'm
a little bit cooler
to everyone,
even myself,
because Mr. Hoeksema
called me
a peach.

A Nap

I toss my backpack on the floor,
shove the extra pillows off the couch,
and lie down.
I'm falling asleep
when Mom says, "Kay."
I imagine her teeth grinding.
I don't even open my eyes.
"Mom, I'm taking a quick nap
before I do my homework."
"Kay, clean this up now.
You know Gran Eula hates her pillows
on the floor."
"I just need a quick nap."
I glare at her.
"It's not like the pillows are getting dirty
or anything."
"Now, Kay.
Get up and fix the couch."
I sit up and shove the pillows back in place.
"Why does everything
have to be so perfect for you?"
I grab my bag and stomp to my room.
"It's not me, young lady. It's Gran Eula."

"Oh, right," I say under my breath.
I stop myself from slamming my bedroom door
and close it instead.
I shove all my pillows off the bed
and flop onto my bedspread.
Anger vibrates
under my skin.

Questions

Tap, tap, tap.
"Come in," I say.
"How about an apology?" says Mom.
"I'm sorry," I mumble.
"Thank you." She sits on the edge of my bed,
scoops my pillows from the floor,
and arranges them along my headboard.
"How was school today?" she asks.
All the anger comes up again.
Like if I tell her, I know she'll say,
"Why did you miss that on the test?"
and
"Why did you choose that topic
for the assignment?"

and
"By the way, I don't like that shirt
with those shoes."
"Shut up already and let me take a nap,"
I want to say.
"Fine," I answer.

So Unbelievable

A little later
Grandma Margie comes in.
She sits on my blow-up chair.
"I love the way
this wobbles me around," she says.
"Me, too."
She rolls and sways
till I start laughing with her.
"Your laugh is exactly like your mother's, Kay."
"Nuh-uh," I say.
"Yes, it is. You two really are so much alike.
That's why you argue."
"That is so unbelievable."
"You'll see when you grow up." She smiles.
"Now, help me out of this contraption."

I pull her up.
The chair whistles air back into itself.
Gran Eula walks past my door.
"Sounds like someone passing a mighty wind
in there!"
Grandma Margie and I
lean against each other
and laugh harder.

Never Ever Hear

How come
I get
Grandma Margie
more than Mom?
And it's easier
even to get
Gran Eula.
Sometimes
it seems
Mom and I could
yell and yell and yell,
if I ever dared,
and we'd never ever hear

each other.
How are we alike?
I don't get it.

Hairdos

Saturday morning,
ten o'clock,
Grandma Margie and I
walk into the salon
and sit down in the comfy, slick gold chairs.
We have our hair
washed,
dried,
and styled.
Even get our nails painted
with Glamour Red frosted polish.
All the smells, from
sweet potpourri
to acidy perm solution,
make me feel totally grown up.
Grandma Margie
winks at me
in the mirror.

Gum

In the Quick Mart
next to the salon,
Grandma Margie
lets me choose a pack of gum.
She pays,
and we walk outside.
"That's the same gum
your dad liked to chew," she says.
"Really?" I push the stick into my mouth.
"Yes. He always seemed
to be working a piece over."
"Huh." I press the crosswalk button.
The traffic rolls past.
"You know, I don't think of him
all that much," I say.
"Hm," she answers.
A car speeds through the yellow light.
"Do you think that's okay?" I ask.
"Sure."
The traffic stops,
and we step into the street.
"He left a long time ago," says Grandma Margie.

"Yeah. It's like he cut himself out of us."
"I can see how you think that," she says.
"Living with your mom,
Gran Eula, and me is normal for you now."
We step up onto the sidewalk
and head toward home.
"There may come a time
when you want to track him down."
I shrug.
"And that could be okay too."
"I guess so," I say. "But it's hard to imagine
ever wanting to."

Decision

How could she decide
on a mastectomy?
How can a doctor cut off
a part of a person, anyway?
Not a lump,
but a whole body part.
And where does the part end up?
Where do they put
all the breasts

87

once they're cut off?
Is there a room
with rows of breasts
lined up,
or do they drop them in garbage bags?
Where do the breast bags go?
How will the doctor know
if he cut off all the cancer?
And how will she look later?
How can we sit eating Gran Eula's scrapple
like nothing's gone crazy?

Nightmare

I burst awake
and feel
my heart
pound
against
my hand
on my chest.

This Morning

I step out the door
and jump back
from the huge crab
on our porch,
claw raised,
stabbing the air,
miles from water.
He's ready to take me on
like a mighty warrior
in trusty armor.
I take a step closer.
He raises his claw higher.
It's a dare.
"All right," I mumble,
and go back inside for a minute
so he can scurry away with dignity.
When I come back out,
he's gone.

Chatter

Who's cute
and who's not
is all my friends
chatter about.

Sure, I think
David's cute,
and sometimes
he sits
next to me on the bus.
That's when he isn't going out
with someone like Cindy
or spending all his time
flirting with Deb
while he traces her
entire body.

But come on,
do we have to
chatter,
chatter,
chatter
about who's cute
constantly?

The Cafeteria

"Mastectomy."
"Oh, man," says Sheray.
"I'd never do that," says Deb.
She swings her hair
forward
until her chest is covered.
"Who would let someone
cut off her whole breast?"
I slam my lunch tray down.
My stupid Tater Tots bounce
across the table.
"Maybe she loves her family
more than herself!" I say.
"Maybe she's willing
to cut off one part
so she doesn't die
and leave us forever."
Everyone near our table
stares.
I walk away
from Deb and Sheray.

In the Crowded Hall

God,
I hope it's right
for Grandma Margie
to get a mastectomy.
If she cuts it off,
if she does her part,
will you make her totally better
forever?
That seems fair, God.
Please?

PE

Coach blows his whistle
and the pack of us
runs.
Slowly
we circle the track,
trying not to sweat buckets
so we don't have to shower.
Trying not to trip,

especially near the boys
on the field.

Coach yells, "Pick it up, ladies!"
That ticks me.
Ticks me so much
I take off.
Faster and faster.
The pack is way behind me.
I lap the track,
once,
twice.
Coach grabs my arm.
"You all right, Kay?" he bellows.
I wrench free
and keep on running.

We Hate It

Everyone
hates showering
naked
in front of everyone else.
I go

as fast as I can,
hardly getting the soap
to lather in my hands.
I slide
the few bubbles
down my legs
and off my toes.
Squeak, squeak.
The knob is hard to turn off.
I grab my towel
and wrap up tight
before everyone
sees
me.

Period

I would have died
if I was Hattie.
She got her period
during science.
A big spot
on the back of her plaid wool skirt.
I would have died

when everyone
pointed and laughed.
"Nice science project," they hooted.
"Enough!" said Ms. Certel.
Hattie
walked
out the door
and didn't come back
till the next day.
Did she cry?
I would have died.

Another Nightmare

Tomorrow
they
are
cutting
off
her
breast.
I flip over.
I'm having a nightmare,
and I haven't even

fallen
asleep yet.

Thmp

"Be brave," says Gran Eula.
"We'll be right here waiting," says Mom.
"We'll be praying, Grandma Margie."
"Thank you," she whispers,
and even manages a smile.

"You ladies
will need to wait out here,"
says the big man nurse.
We nod.
He wheels away Grandma Margie
on the bed.
She's already hooked up
to an IV.

We stand in the hallway
and watch the turquoise doors
swing
thmp, thmp, thmp
to a stop.

Our three shadows
stretch across the pink floor squares.
Three separate gray stripes
trying to reach those doors
but not making it.

The Surgery

I sip cool hot chocolate.
The stupid vending machine
splashed half down the side
of the paper cup.
I lick the bitter powder lumps
off my lips.

The fluorescent lights flicker
off-on-off
above Gran Eula.
She stares straight ahead.

The clock hand jerks
around its pale face
above Mom.
She looks at a magazine
but never turns the pages.

I rub
my runny, burning nose.
This place
stinks.
It's like the formaldehyde we used in science
to preserve the dead mouse we found.
Do doctors use that stuff
to preserve dead bodies
or the cut-off parts
of people?

I try to knit
but keep dropping stitches.

Sip.
Flicker.
Watch.
Knit.

Flicker.
Knit.
Flicker.
Knit.

My knitting
is a giant red knot

lying on my lap.
I need Grandma Margie
to help me
with this mess.
But she's busy
with her own.

Recovery

I can't look
at Grandma Margie's chest.
I try not to look
at all the tubes
going in and out
everywhere.
"Look at this hurking knot," I say
first thing
in recovery.
And it's me who makes
her smile.
All because
my knot is so unbelievably huge.
"We'll untangle this
together,"
she says weakly.

For Her

Seems all I can ever do
is pray
my heart out.
But that's
my part.
They said so.
Grandma Margie did her part
and got her breast cut off.
I hope God
does his part
and makes her better.

Tangy Sweet

"She was up and walking today," says Gran Eula.
"Yes, and her color was better," says Mom.
"That's so great."
I nibble the pickled watermelon rind
Grandma Margie preserved last summer.
The tangy sweet
gives me a tingly chill.
This is so good

I want to tell her.
But she isn't here.

Aren't Saying It

"I'm glad your grandma
is doing okay," says Sheray.
"Thanks."
She moves past to get off the bus.
"Me, too," says Deb.
I nod.
But I know what you said, Deb.
You
could never cut off your breast.
I know
you
think less of my grandma,
even though
you
aren't saying it.
Deb walks past and gets off.
I know what
you're
thinking.

She's Home

It's crazy
how you can have a giant surgery,
then get back home
so soon.
Mom and Gran Eula
pick Grandma Margie up
while I'm at school.
I come home,
and there she is
in her chair.
"You're home!" I shout.
"It's good to be here." She smiles.
"Give me a peck on the cheek, Kay.
I'm not quite up for a hug."
I press my lips to her face.
She smells hospitally still,
but
she's home!

The Two of Them

"These should be lined up
along the counter
so we don't overlook any medicine," says Mom.
She pushes the bottles around.
"They should be
in alphabetical order
so we can find what we need," says Gran Eula.
She pushes the bottles around.
"We could set them on a tray
so they are contained in one place."
Mom digs through
the drawer of pans.
"And we need a sheet of paper
to record when she takes what."
Gran Eula gets a pad
off Mom's desk.
While they arrange the pills
in perfect order,
I squeeze by and get the two aspirin
Grandma Margie has asked for.

Order

Order has always been what
Gran Eula loves most.
Mom learned everything
about being perfect
from her grandma.
And maybe
I've learned a lot
from Grandma Margie.
But what's so big
about order, anyway?
When I was little,
Gran Eula
made my stuffed animals
sit up straight.
Now she puts my CDs
and books
in alphabetical order.
I'm surprised
Gran Eula
didn't command
Grandma Margie's cancer cells
to march right out of her body
in an orderly,

systematic
fashion.
Mom would have probably
tallied up the numbers
and made a spreadsheet
or something.

The Recovery

When Mom cleans Grandma Margie's stitches,
I sit in the living room
so I don't see anything.
Gran Eula gives her full attention
to cooking eggplant parmesan.
I cross my legs up on the couch
and wonder
if the surgeon
will cut off
one of my breasts
one day.

Super Serious

Since the surgery
we act super serious.
Even when Mom and I bowl,
it's like
we are in a tournament
or something.
We check the screen
to see our score
constantly.
We pause longer
before we throw the ball.
We don't buy
curly cheese fries or soda.
So when I see David
three lanes over
and wave and smile,
guilt
gushes into my stomach
like I've betrayed Grandma Margie.
"Who's that?" Mom asks.
"Just David."
"Oh, he's cute," she teases.
"Mom, shhhh!" I giggle.

Our seriousness
is broken
at least for this second.

Hug

"I'm feeling better, Kay,"
says Grandma Margie.
"Give me a hug."

I'm so scared
I'll feel it missing.
I'll squeeze too hard.
I'll hurt her.
Some last bit of cancer will
jump into me.
I'm so scared
of this hug.

I feel the sick, empty spot
where her breast used to be,
but Grandma Margie
is behind it.

They All

At church they all
are so nice.
Miss Martha Faye asks,
"How's she doing?"
"Good," I say.

"How are you doing?"
asks the lady in the pew behind us.
"Fine."

"What have you been doing?"
asks our pastor.
"The normal stuff."

Their questions make me wonder
if I am fine.
Am I acting normal?
I just want to get home
and make sure
Grandma Margie really is
doing all right.

Time

It takes time to get better.
Mom helps with the painful exercises
to stretch Grandma Margie's
stitched muscles.
During an arm lift Mom asks,
"Finished your homework, Kay?"
"Yes," I say.
It's funny
Mom has to mother
her mother
and me.

Gran Eula cooks chicken livers
to increase the iron
in Grandma Margie's blood.
"Clear your plates, you three," she says at dinner.
She's mothering
all of us.

I make sure Grandma Margie's water bottle
stays full to help her gain strength.
I'm doing it too.

The three of us are mothering,
but Grandma Margie is still healing
slowly.

It seems like when the surgeon cut away
her breast,
some of her life
leaked out too.

Friends

I read
in the empty time.
I read at doctors' offices.
I read after nightmares.
I read when I hide out in the bathroom
and rest my head against the toilet paper roll.
I turn page after page,
in book after book.
Other kids
suffer in novels.
I'm not the only one.
My stuff
could be worse.

I hold the open book to my face
and breathe deep.
The ink paper smell
fills me up.
Each author
is a friend saying,
"There's hope.
Look."

"Hit the Showers, Ladies"

"I'm too skinny."
"I'm too fat."
"My thighs are too big."
"My chest is too small."
Idiots!
For the first time
I'm not ashamed
of how I look
when I shower
after PE.
I have
all my body parts,
and none of them

are sick
with cancer.
Who cares
what shape
everything is
if it's healthy?
I'm alive,
aren't I?

Her Friends

Grandma Margie's friends from prayer group
stop by for iced tea and powdered lime cookies.
But really,
who cares about:
 Patty Sue's ingrown toenail,
 Bob's new mower,
 Imogene's bad haircut,
 Dorcus's daughter's allergies,
 and Joe Bob's trip to Sanibel?
"How nice," says Grandma Margie,
and, "Is that so?"
I don't think Grandma Margie
really cares.

She seems so tired
when they leave.
But they seem happy.
Their duty is finished.

Warrior

I call Grandma Margie "Warrior"
because Mr. Hoeksema said
Spartan women
used to cut off a breast
to be better archers.
Grandma Margie says
she's not ready to pick up
a bow and arrow,
but I still call her
"my warrior."

On the Way to the Diner

We drive by David
mowing his lawn.
"David!" I say aloud,
not meaning to.
"Now, he's the cat's meow,"
says Gran Eula.
"No wonder you're blushing.
He is the bee's knees, all right."
Mom and Grandma Margie
are talking up front,
so they don't hear,
but I'm still
so, so embarrassed,
until Gran Eula
finally says,
"Now, now, sugarplum."
She digs out a roll of candy
from her pocketbook
and pinches me off
a green one,
which means
"Don't worry.
Blushing

is perfectly
okay."

One Evening

No, I don't want to see.
"Okay," I say.

No, I don't want to see!
"She wants to see," Mom tells Grandma Margie.

No, I don't want to see!!
Grandma Margie turns around
and opens her robe at the top.

No, I don't want to see:
the jagged red line,
the silver staples,
the blue sutures tied in little knots,
and the queer, empty spot
of pasty skin.

"That's not so bad, Grandma Margie."
I'll never
ever

forget
seeing
this horribleness.

Mean

Today
some girls
hide Hattie's clothes
when she's in the shower.
Deb and Sheray laugh.
I do too.
"Come on, Kay,"
they call.
"I'll catch up in a minute."
When everyone else leaves,
I dig Hattie's clothes out of the garbage.
I am late for my next class,
but Hattie mutters, "Thanks."

Squeezed

I squeeze my homework
in
when I can.
In study hall,
at lunch,
in between helping Grandma Margie.
I'm doing homework,
but I'm slipping
behind.

Wiggly Jiggly Prostheses

Mom holds the store door open.
"You'll feel better wearing one,"
she tells Grandma Margie.
"With or without is fine," says Gran Eula,
"but don't ask me to feel it."
We walk inside.
Grandma Margie finally says,
"All right. I'll try one."
I check out all the different kinds
of fake breasts

in the showcase.
"Never seen so many bosoms," says Gran Eula.
I get busy
squeezing the squishiness,
jiggling the wiggliness,
until I find the right one
to match Grandma Margie
and fill
her empty space.

Two Bumps

"How do I look? Okay?" asks Grandma Margie.
She faces us,
then turns a bit
so we can check her out.
"Is it comfortable?" asks Gran Eula.
"Sort of," says Grandma Margie.
"It looks completely natural," says Mom.
But
what if it slips?
Slips right out
and falls into her lap,
at church,

or at the diner,
or when my friends are around?
Mom nudges me.
"Your bumps match, Grandma Margie," I blurt.
And we all
end up
giggling.

Sleepover

Deb and Sheray
come over.
"Wait here," I tell them.
Everyone's asleep.
I sneak Grandma Margie's prosthesis
out to show.

"Ooo, let me try it on," says Deb.
"I want to see how I look."
"No." I grab it back and brush it off.
"It's Grandma Margie's.
But you can touch it, Sheray," I say.
"Uh-uh." She shakes her head.
"Come on. There's nothing wrong with it."

I hold it out.
She backs away.
"Fine." I pull it close.
What does she think,
it has cancer cells on it
or something?

"Just wait here," I hiss,
and sneak it
to Grandma Margie's room.
I come back and pretend to go to sleep
while my two friends
whisper.

Just in Case

It's only been a while
since the mastectomy,
but the doctors say,
"Just in case."

Just in case
a speck
is still there.
Even

a
miniscule
dot
of
cancer
has to be
annihilated.

Radiation.
Chemo.

Just in case
it
is still
living
in
Grandma Margie.

The Roach

I saw it scuttle
into the linen closet.
Its hairy leg stuck out
for a second,
then nipped away.

It's lived
through
the Roach Man's
poison.
Easily.

Radiation

Black *x*s,
red *o*s,
tic-tac-toe
where
radiation
goes.

Tired

"Wake up, Grandma Margie," I whisper.
"Time for our walk."
She rolls over
and goes right back
to sleep.
I guess I'll practice my knitting

instead.
It's broiling hot outside anyway.
Rustle, crinkle.
I dig through my plastic bag full of yarn.
Shhhh, click, click, shhhh go my needles.
Grandma Margie
doesn't stir
no matter how much racket
I make.

The Waiting Room

Gran Eula hates it
that chemo
is down
in the hospital's basement.
"How can anyone recover
down
in a hole?"
I look around
at the bald heads
and bony bodies
propped in hard plastic
pea green chairs

beneath glaring fluorescent lights.
Gran Eula's right.
No one
looks like
they're recovering
down
here.

Chemo

The technician
helps Grandma Margie
onto the bed.
"It's nice you can come
and help your grandmother."
She smiles at me.
I try not to stare at her too-tight white uniform
stretched over her big breasts.
What a person
to help women
who've had theirs cut off.
"It is nice of her, isn't it?" says Grandma Margie.
"Since her mother works,
we make my appointments

after school
so Kay can help."
"Yeah. And Gran Eula drives us.
But she likes to stay
out of the way
in the waiting room."
"I understand," says the tech.
"Okay. Let's give this a try.
Sometimes
there's no hair loss
with chemo
if we use ice."
I help pack it
around Grandma Margie's head.
She's trembling.
I tuck her blankets
and hold her hand.
What if
her hair still falls out?
My grandma
has always been particular
about each strand,
the same color as mine.

Between Treatments

Mom cleans up her vomit.
Gran Eula heats hibiscus tea.
I help Grandma Margie back to bed and
blot her clammy forehead
gently.

Hiding

It's easy to hide out
at Deb's house
if Grandma Margie
doesn't have an appointment.
Not go home.
Stay in my world of
school,
friends,
and homework.

We've been working
on our science project.
"These look so great," says Sheray.
"Yeah."

I re-cap my marker.
"But did you notice
you and I always end up in the kitchen working,
and Deb and David get the living room?"
"Well, we can switch whenever," she says.
I nod.
We can,
but I notice we don't
ever.
It's still better
hanging out here, though.

Eventually
I have to go home.
And I can tell
when Grandma Margie says,
"Kay, I'm glad you're finally here,"
that I've hurt her feelings
staying away so long.
Like it's personal.

It is.

A Whole Lot Harder

Ms. Certel
asks me to wait.
"Oooooh! In trouble," someone says.
The class pushes
out the door for lunch.
Ms. Certel leans against her desk.
"Kay, you did poorly on your Elements test.
Why are your grades slipping?"
I don't want to answer and let her know
how hard everything is right now.
"Kay?"
"My grandma's getting over cancer," I squeak.
I put my head down on the cool black tabletop.
I want to float away.
But Ms. Certel pats my back
and holds me down on the planet
until I can reattach myself
and sit up.

"Don't you worry about those grades."
She smiles.
"You spend time with your grandma.
The grades will work out."

I gather my books
and swallow to keep from crying.

Being with Grandma Margie
is a whole lot harder
than making good grades.
I'm failing both.

Eat

"Will you eat?" I ask.
She shakes her head.

"Can you eat?" asks Mom.
She shakes her head.

"Eat!" says Gran Eula,
and Grandma Margie takes a bite.

I guess you have to
always
listen to your mom.

Pep Rally

Clubs.
Cheerleaders.
Sports teams.
Everyone joins
something
and then cheers
about their choice
to make everyone else
believe they're cool
because they fit in.
So how about
the Cancer Club?
That's what I belong to.
Rah, rah, rah.

Weeks

Weeks of radiation,
weeks of chemotherapy,
starting-stopping-starting,
weeks and weeks
for a possible

speck of cancer
that might not
even
be there.

Up with Grandma Margie Last Night

We didn't sleep.
Now I'm
hurrying,
hurrying to class,
backpack tugging
my shoulders
down.
Sweat rolling
into my eyes.
Hurrying before
the bell
blares.
Hoping I don't
fall asleep
in Homeroom.

Outside

Deb and Sheray
are together
without me
a lot.
Walking in the halls,
whispering in study hall,
and finishing up lunch
when I sit down.
"Hey," they say,
then go dump their trays
and leave.
Is it them
pushing me away,
or me pushing them?
Whatever,
I'm on the outside
of where
they're at.

Health

All us girls
sit looking
at the pink pamphlets
on self-examination
for breast cancer.
Everyone giggles,
Deb and Sheray loudest,
but I know
I'll do this craziness
every single month
for the rest of my life,
because now
I'm afraid.
Too afraid
not to.

Aware

Before,
did I ever
really fit in,
before Grandma Margie's cancer?

Now it's like
I have to say the truth
before time runs out.
I'm not in any group,
and I'm not going out
with any guy.
Everyone still treats me okay,
but I'm not in
with the kids who hang out
under the flagpole,
or even with Deb and Sheray.
Not like before.
We started talking less and less,
and now
it doesn't seem like
we talk anymore.
Is it bad
that I don't feel too bad
about it?

The Door Bell

Ding dong.
I forgot my key
so I have to ring
the bell.

Ding dong.
Grandma Margie opens the door,
bent over and shivering;
she lets me in.
"Hi, Kay," she says.
"Hi."

I kick the couch
as I walk by
so Mom wakes.
Why isn't she
at her computer
working?

We both help Grandma Margie
settle in her chair.
"Sorry," we say
to Grandma Margie.

"How could you
forget your key, Kay?" Mom whispers.
"How could you
take a nap?" I hiss back.
I flinch from Mom's look.

We pile blankets on Grandma Margie
even though
we
are boiling hot.

Pick, Pick

Some guy
slams into Hattie in the hall.
Her books crash to the floor.
He high-fives another kid,
and they walk away.
Hattie picks up her stuff.
She puts up with so much,
without one friend.
Pick, pick, pick.
They never let up
picking

on her
just like
a cancer.

Art

I'm reaching into the drying rack
for my papier-mâché mask
and brush a roach
with my hand.
I jump,
and it scurries off,
leaving behind
a big hole
where it nibbled
through the forehead.
The class is laughing at David
playing air guitar with his paintbrush.
So no one saw how
I touched the roach,
how
I jumped,
and how
the roach picked

my mask to eat.
No one saw,
because I buried my mask
in the garbage
under a mound of brown paper towels.
I plunge some newspaper strips
into the blobby gunk
to make a new mask.
But I still know
the roach
picked
me.

Less

Less medicine.
More food.
Less hair.
Less hair.
Less hair.
More strength.
Less is more.

Shave It

"Might as well
shave it," says Grandma Margie.
"I can't stand it
half there and half not.
I'll wear a bandanna
till it grows back."
"I can't do it," I say.
"Me, either," says Mom.
Gran Eula wets the razor
and shaves
her daughter bald.

Dinner

I mention Hattie at dinner.
How everyone makes fun of her
and how she doesn't fit in.
"She's the last one on the bus
and always sits in the empty seat
behind the driver.
No one else
ever sits there."

"That is sad," says Mom.
"But it can still be okay not to fit in.
I never did."
"Me, either," says Gran Eula.
"Well, I used to," says Grandma Margie,
sitting there bald.
"Do you fit in?" asks Mom.
I flick a black-eyed pea
to the center of my plate.
"Not really.
I kind of move around
from one group to another."
"Kay, it's all right
not to fit in," says Mom.
But is it all right
for me?

Does It Matter?

"You recall
I only got to the sixth grade."
"Yes, Gran Eula." I've heard it a million times.
"I had to work in the cotton fields
with my parents."

"Uh-huh."
"My friends
walked past our fields
on their way to the schoolhouse.
Walked right past me and my sack.
They always laughed and pointed."
I look down. "I never knew that part."
"Well, now you do.
And you can see,
I did not
fit in."

"And I used to beat
every boy on the block
at every game,"
Mom says, wiping the sweat
off her iced tea
with a napkin.
"That's one way
to not have friends.
Beat the boys.
They don't like you,
and then the girls can't stand you either,
for some crazy reason."
She downs the rest of her drink.

"I did not fit in."
"Wow," I say.

"Well, I did," says Grandma Margie.
"I went to the parties,
and cotillion,
and football games.
I always had a boy on my arm."
She stares at the hibiscus flowers
in the vase.

"But look at us now, Kay."
She folds her napkin carefully.
"Does any of that
matter now?"

Gran Eula, one eyebrow raised—
tough and serious.
Grandma Margie, scratching her scalp—
brave and strong.
Mom, tucking her hair behind her ear—
still good at stuff.
"Nope."

Clean

"Clean" is what they call it.
Grandma Margie is clean of cancer.
We call it
"Time to Celebrate."
Gran Eula fries some okra and catfish.
Mom squeezes fresh limeade.
I turn up my CD
and make everyone dance,
even Gran Eula.

Grandma Margie's clean!
Grandma Margie's clean!
Grandma Margie's clean!

What's Best

Thank you, God,
for doing what's best,
cleaning the cancer
out of Grandma Margie.
Thanks
for doing that.

Pre-algebra Now

X can only be one number.
Y can only be one number
for the perfect equation.
If x is Grandma Margie,
and y is health,
then the perfect equation
equals
life.

To Finish

"And then
you bind off loosely," says Grandma Margie.
She knits back over my last row,
catching one stitch over another.
"I see."
"Then slip the last stitch off and
thread your yarn through the hole."
"It's like a knot," I say.
"Mm-hmm."
She snips my knitting
from the yarn ball.

"What about this piece hanging like a tail?"
"You weave and tuck that on the back side
with a crochet hook
until it disappears."
"Okay."
The string gets shorter and shorter,
until it's gone.
Grandma Margie hands me my knitting.
I pry between the stitches to see the buried yarn.
There is the tippy end
tucked deep inside.
All the threads are loose
and fanning apart
where she cut it.
"It won't unravel?" I ask.
"No. It's wrapped in there tight."
I run my hand
over my big purple square.
"Why don't we put this
over the back of the couch?" she says.
"Okay." I smooth it out.
"That's beautiful," says Grandma Margie.
"Thanks," I say.
It is.

Gin

Gran Eula is fierce
playing gin.
She picks up
a huge row,
and I smile.
"Hold your horses," she growls.
I'm about busting up
waiting for her to organize
her hand.
"Rummy," I say
in two plays,
dropping my last card.
I'm ready to duck
because Gran Eula's shoe
sometimes gets thrown
across the room
when she loses.
But today she smiles back and says,
"You are getting better."
I know it.

Unloading

"Here."
I take the small plates
from Mom.
She unloads the big ones
from the dishwasher.
I restack the small ones
off-center
on purpose.
She nudges them over.
"Here."
I take the cups
and nudge the small plates again.
"Would you stop?" She laughs
and moves them back.
"Well, you can't," I say.
"Can't what?"
"Can't leave those plates off-center."
"That's ridiculous." She closes the cupboard.
I open it, move them again,
and close it.
We cross our arms,
start to giggle,
then bend over laughing.

But Mom still has to open the cupboard
and set things straight.
"Oh, dear." She laughs.
"You're right."

Taking Our Walk

Grandma Margie slips off her bandanna.
"Do you see it?"
"Yep," I say, squinting in the sun
at Grandma Margie's pale peach fuzz
standing on end
all over her head.
I don't care if the neighborhood
sees.
What is better
than a walk
to the canal to fish
in the warm sun
with my Grandma Margie
and her peach fuzz?

Again

We are laughing
again,
at jokes,
at the TV,
at *M*★*A*★*S*★*H*,
at each other.
We are willing
and looking
to laugh
at just about
everything.

Right Now

"And she smiled
at the ice cream man," says Gran Eula.
"No!"
"Yes!"
"With your false teeth
over her own?" I howl.
"Yes, ma'am."
"Well, I was only five," says Mom.

Grandma Margie clutches her waist.
"Oooh," she laughs. "I have a stitch in my side."
"That's better than the ones you had
after surgery," I say.
And for some reason
that is absolutely hilarious
to us
right now.

Vacation

"Bye," everyone calls
at each bus stop.
"Have a good Thanksgiving."
"Bye, Deb and Sheray." I wave.
They move down the aisle
but look back,
surprised
that I've talked to them.
"Bye," they say,
and get off the bus.
I snuggle down in my seat.
I actually feel happy enough

to try
to be nice.

Thanksgiving

Potato rolls
and collard greens,
creamed corn
and sugar beets,
baby peas
and bread-and-butter pickles,
smoked turkey
and shoo-fly pie,
real whipped cream
and no cancer.
There's a lot of thanksgiving
going on
at this table.

I Call Her

"That's so great about your Grandma Margie,"
says Deb on the phone.
"Yeah."
"Now we can go back to normal," says Deb,
"hanging out and stuff.
And I have to fill you in on everything.
There's so much you've missed."
I start to zone out
on her gossip.
Was everything
really so great before?
"And she said
she liked him,
but he didn't!"
Who cares?
I don't.
Why did I call her?

She Didn't Tell Us

"Karine, it's for you," says Gran Eula.
"Dr. Stevens."
"Doctor?" asks Grandma Margie.
"Stevens?" I ask.
Mom doesn't look at us.
"Yes," she says into the phone.
"Nothing? . . .
Benign," she whispers.

Mom hangs up the phone
and walks out of the room
saying nothing.
"Benign?" we mouth
to each other.

The Nerve

My mother had a lump
or something
and didn't tell
any of us.
So it's benign

this time.
But next time
when will she tell
us?
Next time
do I even want
to know?
I crumple my math homework
and slam it at my bedroom wall.
Yeah, I guess
I want to know
everything
next time.

Mama Mia's Taco Town

I squeeze the package
until my hot sauce blurts out.
"So, what was it?" I ask.
"What?" asks Mom.
"The thing."
"Thing?"
I twist the corner of my napkin
and yank it off.

"The benign thing."
"Oh, that."
She eats a plain nacho chip.
Pats her lips with her napkin.
"It was nothing."
"Nothing?!"
People look over.
"Honey, shh."
"I want to know next time."
"There won't be a next time."
She eats another chip.
Not even a crumb falls.
"So you can say
you'll tell me then."
"Sure, honey."
You just better.
Better not
leave me out.
Or alone.

During a Commercial

"I am still your mother," says Gran Eula.
"I am still your mother," says Grandma Margie.
"I am still your mother," says Mom.
"Okay, okay. I'll go get the fudge pops," I say.

Mom?

"Mom,
where's my backpack?" I holler.
"Mother,
where are my keys?" asks Mom.
"Mother,
where's my sweater?" asks Grandma Margie.
Gran Eula grins
and plays another round of solitaire.

Paint

The black
gloops against my paintbrush.
I drag it down half my mask.

"Black?" asks Christie.
"Just for half."
The paint swirls off my brush
into the water like ribbons.
I squeeze the bristles dry.
The yellow paint
is thick and smooth.
I cover the other half
of my mask.
"That's cool," she says.
"Thanks. I like yours, too."
Hers is totally pink with feathers.
"Mine's called *Fairy Dreams*."
She holds hers up to her face.
"Mine's *Before and After*."
"Before and after what?"
I paint red stitches on the black half.
"Cancer."

Checkups

First checkup
Check
Second checkup

Check
Third checkup

The phone rings.

That Doctor's Fault

It's his fault.
He didn't cut
deeply enough,
far enough,
wide enough,
and it's back,
growing all through
my Grandma Margie.
Not his grandma.

In My Room

I slam my fist
into my pillow.
I kick my bed.

"I did my part.

She did her part.
Why did you stop, God?
This can't be what's best!
Why is the cancer back?"
I hold my burning throat.
The whispers have cut deep.

I curl
onto my bed and groan.
"It doesn't make any sense, God.
Don't you hear me?"

What's Next?

I dry my face on my sleeve
and go to the living room.
They're still planning.
"What'll we do?" I ask.
"We'll consider the options,
then come to a conclusion," says Gran Eula.
"Right. We'll start over again," says Mom.
"Probably begin treatments
around the holidays.
The doctor suggested

between Christmas and New Year's."
Grandma Margie
goes to her room
and shuts her door.
"We have some time
to think about it," says Mom.
Do we?

Breakfast

My cereal clatters
into my bowl.
"What are you reading?"
Grandma Margie
looks up from her Bible.
"'Trust in Jehovah
with all thy heart
and lean not upon thine own
understanding:—'"

"'In all thy ways acknowledge him,
and he will
direct
thy paths.'"

"Very good, Kay."
"I memorized that
ages ago."
"Yes, memorizing
is the easy part.
The hard part
is doing it."
That's for sure.

Crawdad

"Do it," says Carlos.
"Go on." Buff nudges Deb.
I wave my hands, *Don't,*
but Deb looks away.
She sticks the smelly crawdad
we're dissecting
on the rim of Hattie's baseball cap.
"Iiiiick," Hattie squeals, and jumps.
Her papers slip to the floor,
and the crawdad
clatters to the table.
The whole class laughs at her
but me.

Hattie hurries to the sink
and scrubs the formaldehyde
out of her cap.
"What were you thinking?" I whisper to Deb.
She shrugs. "Come on, Kay.
It's only Hattie."
I snatch her papers up,
put them on her notebook,
and set the crawdad in the white bowl.
Sheray gives Deb
a thumbs-up.
I'm not part of their group.
For sure.
I don't want to be.

It's Obvious

I cast on
the yellow yarn.
"That is going to be
a beautiful scarf," says Grandma Margie.
"I hope so."
She finishes another row
of the blue angora blanket

she's working on.
Click, shhh, click, shhh.
Our needles talk back and forth.
Before I can stop it,
the question I've been carrying
bubbles up
and out.
"How come
Gran Eula's healthy,
Mom's healthy,
and I'm healthy,
but you're growing cancer?"
Her fingers don't slow down a bit.
Click, shhh.
"It's the hand
of God."

Figuring It Out

"But I did my part."
"Pray?"
"Mm-hm."
"Good."
"And you did your part."

"The mastectomy?"
"Mm-hm."
"We've done our parts, Kay.
Let it rest."

Church

Feeling badly,
she doesn't come with us,
and they ask how she's doing.
We'd rather talk about something else.

Feeling better,
she does come with us,
and they try not to stare.
We'd rather they look elsewhere.

We just want
to try to worship
as part of the body
and not be the diseased part,
separated by sickness.

The Church Friends I Had

They are nice
on the outside
and don't talk
about Grandma Margie.
But no one saves me
a seat anymore.
Not even Sheray.
She looks down
and pretends to read her notes
from last week's sermon.
Mom says, "It's because
they don't know what to say."
Gran Eula says, "It's because
they are selfish."
So I sit with my family
all around me,
and that helps
a little.

Thinking During the Sermon

Gran Eula's friends Miss Drucilla and Mrs. Adele
usually stay for another glass of tea
after their bridge game is over.

Grandma Margie
calls her friends Orpha and Arnold
every couple of weeks.
Even though they live upstate.

Mom goes shopping
and has dinner out
with Essie, Barbara, and Joan
every now and then.
They've known each other
since high school.

They each have
a couple good friends.
Maybe that's how many
you actually need,
all I might need.

And Hattie
doesn't have

even
one.

During Prayer

Grandma Margie sings
even if she can't stand
through all six verses.

She drinks up the preaching,
never looks away from our pastor.

I know she smiles during prayer,
because I peeked.

Grandma Margie doesn't seem sick at all
when she's worshiping.

The Butt

Hattie's the butt of every joke,
sitting alone at lunch.
"Couldn't get the stain out of your skirt, Hattie?"
"Ooooh. What are you eating, Hattie?"

"What's that smell? Oh, it's Hattie!"
Shut up!
I want to scream.
She's a person, too!
Instead,
I sit down
next to her
at the lunch table.
She's not the butt,
they are.

Hi

"Hi."
"Hi."
We don't
say
much
more,
but Hattie
is smiling
for once.

Winter Break

"Whoohooo!" Carlos yells.
"No school for two weeks," says David.
They jump around
and rock the bus.
"Sit," says the driver.
At each stop
a bunch of kids
shove to get
out the door.
Squeeeeeeak.
Shhhh.
Deb and Sheray's stop.
Deb's backpack
bangs against my arm.
She keeps going.
Doesn't say, "Sorry,"
"Bye,"
or, "Have a good holiday."
Both of them are carrying their
science project drawings.
I haven't seen or thought of mine
since when?
It's still at Deb's,

I guess.
Oh, well.
I can get it back
sometime
and finish it up
somehow.
She and Sheray
get off the bus,
and we pull away.
Their matching Santa hats
get smaller and smaller.
"Whoohooo!" Carlos yells.
"No school!"
"Sit," says the bus driver.

The Usual

"The usual?" the waitress asks.
We nod.
Grandma Margie turns up her cup
for her hot water and instant coffee,
and fingers her short white hair.
I guess she used to dye it
the same color

as mine.
I sip my soda.
The usual
is the only
usual thing
we have left.

Mom's Turn

Last year Gran Eula
got out her artificial tree
that never drops needles.
So this year
it's Mom's turn
for a real tree
with a sharp, piney smell.
I'm glad Grandma Margie
gets to sit and smell
a real tree
this Christmas.

A Gift

A thermometer,
a bottle of antacid,
or a heating pad?
What kind of gift
is loved
by a person
who is sick
like Grandma Margie?

In the Kitchen

"Hand me that spatula, please," says Gran Eula.
"In a minute. I need it," says Mom.
"Well, could you pass the pot holder?"
"No, I need that, too."
I swallow my water
and sneak out of there fast.
With both of them
trying to fix
everything Grandma Margie likes
for Christmas Eve dinner,

the kitchen
is way too hot.

Good Morning

Mom wakes me
on Christmas morning.
"Honey, I want you to know
this is a small Christmas.
Money's tight
because we need to save.
Grandma Margie
will be starting treatments again."
"I know."
I know Mom's worked late nights
to keep our money steady.
I know I fall asleep
to her keyboard clicking.
I know
money is tight.
"It's okay, Mom.
I know."

Christmas

Gifts are opened.
They're small.
CDs.
Socks.
Books.
Grandma Margie gives me
my own knitting needles.
"I love it, Kay." She holds up
the framed photo
of us fishing
for everyone to see.
We eat
the gingerbread men
Gran Eula made for us.
And now we are driving
around the neighborhood
looking at the twinkling lights
on the palm trees
and the plastic pink flamingos
wearing Santa hats.
People sit in their lawn chairs
out front,
drink soda and beer,

and wave.
Everyone's in shorts and T-shirts.
"Merry Christmas."
"Merry Christmas."
We drive on
to oooh and aaah
in harmony
at the lights.

The Beach

Mom takes us
to the beach
in the dark early morning.
Gran Eula sets the gas cookstove
on the picnic table and lights it.
Tssssssss.
The eggs slide over the iron skillet.
She heats up
grits and gravy
by lantern light.
Mom sets the table.
"Don't go far," calls Gran Eula.
Grandma Margie and I walk the surf,

stepping around shifting horseshoe crabs.
The fishy breeze mixes
with the bubbling gravy smell.
The gulls squawk.
We eat in the pale pink light
of the sunrise.
"Mmmm," says Grandma Margie.
The eggs are just runny enough
to slip into the grits.
The gravy is lumpy with bits of sausage.
Everything tastes so good
out here.
Saltier, and smoother.
"You have to wait
a half an hour to swim," says Mom.
"An hour," says Gran Eula.
We head for the warm water
before even the half hour is up.
Just to wade.
"Come on," says Mom.
We dive in.
"All right, you two rascals," calls Gran Eula.
But then
she and Grandma Margie

walk in
till their shoulders are covered.

Race

Mom and I race,
doing the crawl stroke.
I go as far as I can.
"Ugh." I slap the water.
She's still going.
I tread.
Grandma Margie and Gran Eula
hardly make ripples
doing the breaststroke.
Is it still called that
for Grandma Margie?
My feet dangle,
barely touching the sand.
A cold stream of water
slips past my ankle.
I turn over and float
to get closer to shore.
The sun moves
into the blue sky.

When people start showing up,
we pack to leave.
"Brush that sand off your feet," says Gran Eula.
"We are," Mom and I say.
I see some kids I know from school,
but I don't want to stay.
I slip my sand-free feet
back into my flip-flops.
I'm ready
to go home
with my family.

Our Hair

This time
the chemo
makes her hair fall out
fast.

I see Grandma Margie at her dresser mirror
put a chunk of white hair
back up to her forehead
to cover some of her baldness
for a second.

I go put on
my baseball cap.

The Wig

Mom and Gran Eula bring home a wig.
"A late Christmas gift!"
They tease it.
"Oh, it's lovely," says Mom.
Shape it.
"Very natural," says Gran Eula.
And spray it.
"Perfect," they say
to make Grandma Margie feel better.
"It's a little hot." She looks in the mirror.
"And itchy." She scratches under the edge.
"It's worth it," they say.
"Okay."
But after a few days
Grandma Margie buries it in the trash,
when they aren't home,
and ties on her bandanna.
The wig

only made them
feel better.

New Year's Eve

"Gin," says Mom.
Gran Eula swipes up the cards.
"Deal," she says.
Mom grins.

Grandma Margie looks up from her knitting.
"That scarf is looking so nice, Kay."
"Thanks."

Gran Eula
is smirking at Mom.
She must have a good hand
this time.
"I don't think
you'll win this one,
Granddaughter," she says.

I glance up.
Mom and me
are both granddaughters

spending time
with our grandmothers
on New Year's Eve.
Not exactly
the greatest party
with all the cool kids from school,
but
special.

A Whisper

"Good-bye."
"Thank you."
We file out past our pastor
and shake his big hand.
A whisper in my ear says,
"Deb's going out with David."
I turn quick enough
to see Sheray
slip past Mom
and squeeze out the door.
"It's good to see you today, Kay,"
says Pastor.
"Thank you," I mumble.

Gran Eula reaches forward
to shake his hand,
so I don't get to.
Outside
the glaring sunshine
reflects off the white concrete
pavement.
Deb and David?
I shield my eyes
and squint at the milling crowd.
Sheray isn't around.
Deb and David.
She knows how much I like him.
I guess it
doesn't matter
anymore.

Back to School

Back
at
it.
Halls
and

classes
streaming by.
Deb
and
David
holding hands
every
time
I
turn
around.
Back
at
it.

Treatments

Get the vomit bucket.
Get the warmer covers.
Get them off.
Get a clean washcloth.
Get a glass of cool water.
Get the medicine.
Get no sleep.

A Spot

Hattie
doesn't have to
save me a place
at lunch.
The table
is always
empty
around
her.
It's nice to know
there's
a spot
for me.
I set
my tray down.
"Hi." She looks up at me.
"Hi."

Captain Crabs

Mom and I stop for a bucket of garlic crabs
after bowling.
"You need time to relax, Kay," she says.
"You've helped so much with Mother,
and you're constantly under
that homework load."
She stops for a big bite of meat.
I keep eating.
I don't want to talk about the homework
I'm not getting done.

"So, tell me," she says. "How's David?"
"He dumped Cindy,
and now he's going out with Deb."
"Hmmm," says Mom.
"It stinks," I say.
"It does."
She passes me a claw.
I crack it open and tear the meat out.
"Men," we say,
and shrug.

Dad

"Is that the way Dad was?"
"You mean fickle?"
"Yeah."
She lets out a big sigh.
"I guess you could say that.
He was fickle enough to leave."
I lick the grease
off my fingers.
"Are you glad?"
She wipes her hands
on a napkin.
"No. I loved him."
"From the little bit I remember,
I guess I did too." I look down.
"It'd be kind of nice
to know how we are alike
and stuff. Or just see
who he is now."
"I can understand that, hon.
If you ever want to find him,
I'd be happy to help you."
"Thanks." I look up. "But I don't feel like
doing that right now."

"Okay."
I run my finger
around the bottom of the bucket
and lick off all the garlic bits.
Mom smiles.
"What?" I say.
"Your father used to do
the same thing."
Huh.

Why Him?

I roll over in bed.
Why did I ever like David?
Well, he's cute
and has a great smile,
with that little chip in his tooth
so he looks
tough.
I fluff my pillow.
But what about
how he goes from girl to girl?
That stinks.

My head sinks
into the feathers.
And now even Deb?
What kind of character
does he have, then?
Oh, man.
I roll over.
I sound
like Gran Eula.

Whisperings

Mom and Gran Eula
whisper in the hallway:
"She's not getting better."
"She's losing strength."
"Insurance won't pay."
"How much longer?"
I hate those whispers
that scream
over and over,
louder and louder,
in my brain.

Late

The wind tears at the royal palms.
The fronds finger the black sky
like they are scratching an old chalkboard.
Heat lightning
snaps behind the palmetto field
by the goalposts.
I missed the bus
to school
because I overslept.
Gran Eula, Grandma Margie, and Mom
were finally asleep when I left.
Grandma Margie stopped throwing up
around four o'clock.
But I didn't get to sleep
until five or so.
A fat raindrop
the shape of a ball
splashes open
on my forehead
and runs down.
At least no one
will be able to tell
I've been crying.

The Empty Hall

Squeak, slap.
My sneakers suck
the hallway linoleum.
I stop.
Heavy rain
thumps the roof.
Lightning
cracks
by the window.
The lights go out.
I panic, reach for the wall,
and stub my fingers.
The lights come back on.

I'm still here.
I rub my jammed fingers.

Squeak, slap,
squeak, slap.

For Keeps

Every time
the thunder bangs,
the class cheers
for the lights to go out for keeps.
But I'm sitting here
totally soaked.
My bangs
drip spots
onto my notebook.
I'm the only one
not cheering.
I'm shivering.
Because I don't
want to go home
early.

Nuts

Mom slams down
a bottle of Grandma Margie's medicine.
"I can't believe
it's going to take two days

for the pharmacy to refill this."
She rubs her forehead.
Her hair
swings forward into her face.
It is driving her nuts
she's not perfect enough
to fix Grandma Margie.

Locked

Ugh!
I can't remember
my locker combination.
The dial ridges
roll under my fingers,
round and round.
Numbers stream past.
Kids in the hall
gather
and point
and laugh,
while I spin the dial for hours
because I'm too embarrassed
to ask for help.

I can't stand it another second.
I cry out
and wake up.

Shopping with Mom

Mom waits outside the dressing room
while I try on bathing suits.
There are four naked legs
in the next stall.
A mother and daughter
laugh hysterically
over how bad a bikini looks.
I step out for Mom to see
the striped tankini.
I tug the top
to cover more.
It's like my breasts
are showing
too much.
I don't want to look big
or anything.
Big could mean
there's cancer in there

or something.
I tug at it again.
"Leave it alone, Kay. That's really cute," she says.
"All right."
I cross my arms
over my chest
and go back to the stall.
The other girl steps out.
Her mother's carrying
an armload of suits.
"Let's go look again," she chuckles.
I shut the door.
So what if this bathing suit looks fine on me?
I'm jealous
of that other girl
laughing with her mother.

The Keys

Grandma Margie is up
for a little break.
We head down
to the Keys
for the weekend.

The breeze
licks away our sweat.

Mom does swan dives
off the board.
Grandma Margie sits poolside in a muumuu
with her legs dipped in.
Gran Eula plays solitaire
under the umbrella.
"Ouch, ouch!"
The frying-hot asphalt burns my feet.
I race
to the hotter sand
and jump into the ocean.
My feet cool.
I swim out to the small sandbar
and sit in front of
the sunset.

Purple.
Orange.
Red.
It's so enormous,
so beautiful,
and
I

am
so small.

The Deli

Riding to school,
I notice a new restaurant has opened
on the corner
of Franjo and Caribbean Boulevard.
Right away
I claim it mine.
I'm not going to tell anyone at home
about it.
It'll be my own place
where I can go
and pretend everything is okay.
Like I used to do
at Deb's.
After school
I scrounge a few dollars
and walk the couple blocks
to sit down
in a room
with people

who are all normal.
Their talk
presses into me.
I munch my salty kosher pickle
and pretend
to be normal
too.

The Lessons Continue

Sitting beside me,
Grandma Margie teaches me
to read a knitting pattern.
"And this means,
ohh,
well, it means . . ."
The instructions shake
between her fingers.
"I just don't have time
to teach you all this."
"I have time, Grandma Margie."
I don't mention my unfinished homework.
I'll work on it later.
"It's not my bedtime yet.

Go ahead."
But she sits there,
and everything slips from her lap.
"I'm sorry, Kay." She bends and gathers the
papers, yarn, and needles.
I stare at her small, curved back
and sharply
suck in a mouthful of air.
She means
she doesn't have enough
time left.

Floating

Some days
it seems like
I am floating through school
from one place to another.
One class done,
down the hall to the next.
I don't hear anyone,
look at anyone,

or talk to anyone.

I'm the only one
floating
except Hattie.
I see her.
She silently floats by.
It is totally
unreal.

Do You?

Do you float
when you're dead?
From here to there?
Will Grandma Margie float
away?
If she dies?
Am I near dying,
since I'm floating
everywhere?

Blah, Blah, Blah

Their mouths move,
but I hardly understand
what they're saying.
Every one of my teachers
is speaking a foreign language.
Sometimes an English sentence breaks through.
"Singular verb forms end in *s*."
"It's a mixture, not a compound."
"Pick it up, ladies!"
But all the rest is
"Blah, blah, blah."

Out-a-towners

Those out-a-towners
call to ask
if it'd be okay
for them
to stop in for a visit.
Folks Grandma Margie hasn't seen in years
that used to be friends with Grandpa.
"That'd be fine," she says into the phone.

"Want to come and gawk,"
whispers Gran Eula to Mom.
So we help Grandma Margie dress,
pick out a big sun hat,
and do her make-up.
"Margie!" they gush,
and hand over a hurking flower arrangement.
She goes real pale for a second
but then says, "Thank you."
She smiles through the meal
and sips her instant coffee,
while they eat their fried chicken,
lick their greasy fingers,
and stare.
After they leave,
she throws up,
pulls on her pajamas,
and goes straight to bed.
But they'll never know,
those out-a-towners.

The Bouquet

Lilies, carnations, and roses.
My mom smashes them into the garbage
as soon as those guests leave.
Crams them down with her foot.
"Heathens," hisses Gran Eula.
What were they thinking
bringing my Grandma Margie
flowers
left over
from a funeral?

Practice

I read the pattern
and knit
and knit
and knit.
She picks up my dropped stitch.
I knit
and knit
and knit.
She helps me cast off

and bury the ends.
I wrap
and wrap
and wrap
my soft yellow scarf
around
her thin, cold shoulders.
I got it done
in time.

By Accident

Sitting in the deli,
I can't believe
how many people
touch each other,
squeeze a shoulder,
or a hand.
The pretty woman pats
the tired-looking man's back.
The little girl with the braids
kisses her mom's cheek.
The grandma
ruffles the boy's red hair.

It's so strange.
Grandma Margie and I
touch sometimes,
but other than that,
my family doesn't touch,
unless by accident.
Then we say,
"Sorry."

Running

It's running
faster than she breathes.
It's running
to her nodes,
through her blood,
to nest in her bones,
and no one
can stop it.

Sorry

"Sorry," says the doctor.
"Sorry," say the neighbors.
"Sorry," says the church.
"You're sorry!" I yell into my pillow.
I'm sick
of their "sorry's."
"Why?" I muffle my cries.
Why can't anybody
do something
to help her?
I squeeze my pillow tighter
and rock
on my bed.

Nope

When the doctor
offers Grandma Margie marijuana,
she says, "No."
He says, "It will make you feel better."
"Not as long
as I have a granddaughter," she tells him.

"But it helps with the nausea," he states.
She turns away.
My grandma won't smoke pot
because of me.

No One

No one calls
or comes over.
I find my science project drawing
on our porch.
There's still a ton to do.
It seems like years ago
we were all working together at Deb's.
Did she or Sheray
drop it here for me?
Of course whoever it was
didn't knock
and say hi.
They can't talk to me.
They can't risk
slipping
back into my life—
my nightmare.

The Mind Readers

Mr. Hoeksema holds up a card
so we all can see
but David can't.
It has a triangle on it.
"Triangle," says David.
"Oooooh," we say.
"Square," he says.
"Man."
"This one's hard," says David.
We hold our breath.
"Um . . ."
Mr. Hoeksema holds the card steady.
"Circle," says David.
One shiver runs through us all.
"Hey," shouts Christie.
"Mr. Hoeksema is tapping David's foot
to tell him the shape!"
Everyone busts up
over how they've fooled us.
I bite my lip and look away.
I wanted to believe
so bad
that Mr. Hoeksema and David could read minds,

because maybe then
they'd read mine
and I wouldn't be
alone.
David rubs Deb's back.
Well,
maybe if
just Mr. Hoeksema
could read my mind.

Bizarro

Even if Hattie
wanted to come over,
I wouldn't
want her
to smell
the sickness,
thick in our house.
Besides,
Grandma Margie's hospital bed
came today.
It's not like you can miss it.

We put it in the living room
so she can lie down
and still feel part of everything.
Mom works on her accounts
right at the head of the bed.
Grandma Margie says
the clicking keyboard
doesn't bother her at all.
But the whole thing
is bizarro
to me.
Even if Hattie came,
I wouldn't let
her in.

Study Hall Rethought

Study hall
is such a joke.
Who likes who?
Who's going out?
Who's dumped who?
Doesn't anyone know

it's all about
who is going to die
before who?

"How Are You?"

Doesn't Mom get it?
When I say,
"I'm fine,"
it means
I'm not,
and I want to
scream my head off.
Why can't she see
how I really feel?
Why do I say
I'm fine?
So she can feel good
that she has something
under control?
Me?
Why can't she really ask me
and wait for the answer?
However long it takes me

to tell the truth.
Why doesn't she check and see
I'm freaking out?
It's all her fault
she doesn't get
me.

Shortness

It's bad.
Everything is bad.
Gran Eula's short with Mom.
"Karine, don't you go
getting yourself in a pucker!"
Mom's short with me.
"Kay, get this pigsty cleaned up now!"
I slam the pots and pans into their drawers.
Everyone's tired
from taking care of Grandma Margie.
She rolls over and faces the wall.
She must be tired
of us.

Faithful

Grandma Margie
doesn't want her prayer group
to visit anymore.
"I'm not strong enough, Karine."
"It's okay."
"I don't want them to see me like this, Mother."
"I understand," says Gran Eula.
"They can still pray for me, Kay," she says.
"Right."
"But I'd like Pastor
to stop in still."
"Sure," we say.
He comes to visit often,
sits on the stool
next to her bed,
and holds her hand.
He talks with Grandma Margie,
listens to Grandma Margie,
and prays with Grandma Margie.
I hide out in my room,
feeling faithless
in the middle of their faith.

Afraid

"Aren't you afraid?" I ask.
"Of what?" Grandma Margie
sets her Bible aside,
and takes a pill
and glass of water from me.
"Well, like, you know."
I tuck her sheet under the mattress.
"Being so sick and all."
Grandma Margie licks her dry lips.
"I was just reading in Isaiah,
and he says, 'In the shadow
of his hand
he hath hid me.'"
"What does that mean?"
"God is holding me safe."
"But"—I pick at a thread
dangling from her sheet—
"I still don't get
why God thinks
making you sick is best."
I twist the thread until it breaks off.
Grandma Margie covers my hand.
"We don't need to question

what he's doing, Kay.
The shadow of his hand
is the only safe place to be."
"Even if it hurts?"
"Even if it hurts."
She swallows her pain pill,
hands me the empty glass,
and closes her eyes.
"I'm praying for you,"
she whispers.

Now

Sometimes
in the night
when she shakes,
pukes,
and groans,
I pray,
"Please make her die, God.
Now.
It's best."
And in the morning,
when she smiles at me,

I go cry
in shame
that I ever prayed
such a thing.

Hattie

I sit in the front seat on the bus,
behind the driver.
She slides quietly in next to me.
She doesn't say much.
She doesn't ask.
After school
she doesn't call.
She doesn't come over.
She's not afraid of silence.
I sit in the front seat,
and she slides in next to me.
That's enough.

Evening Walk

The doctor suggested
fresh air.
So Gran Eula rented a wheelchair
because Grandma Margie
can only walk
as far as the bathroom.
My flip-flops pat the sidewalk.
Mom pushes the wheelchair.
Grandma Margie's slumped in the seat.
Gran Eula clutches her pocketbook
and sets the pace,
making it clear to the neighbors
we aren't out for a talk,
just a walk
to get us where we're going,
once around the block.

Checking

When we get home,
I check all the closets
and under all the beds
for Grandma Margie.
She can't be still
till I come and tell her
there are no burglars hiding.
I feel stupid looking
and am tempted to not look and to lie instead,
but it's one thing I can do
to give her some peace.
I do it.

Why?

"Why is Grandma Margie
so scared
after we've been out?" I ask Gran Eula.
Ssccccrrrr.
She pulls the lawn chair
across the porch to me.
"Well"—she settles into the seat—

"when she was little,
she walked in on a burglary."
"Really?"
"Yes, ma'am. The burglar
ran when he saw her."
"Whoa. That's creepy."
I rub my cool arms.
"Did he steal a bunch of stuff?"
"Oh, yes." Grandma crosses her legs.
"Let me tell you.
Your Great Grandpa Grant
was furious."

"It's funny," I say, "that Grandma Margie
is so afraid
of seeing another burglar,
but she doesn't seem
all that afraid of being sick."
Gran Eula swallows and looks up
at the first star.

"Sometimes
what we believe
doesn't control
what we do."
"What do you mean?" I lean closer.

"She believes God is sovereign
over everything,
but
she still has to check under our beds."
"That's just because
of what happened to her," I say.
"Right.
For a moment
she forgets
her God
is greater than a burglar."

Wow.
Do I believe stuff
and forget?

Touching

Mr. Hoeksema
patted me on the back
for no real reason.
Ms. Certel
put her arm around my shoulder
and said,

"Hang in there,"
when I was heading out of class.
Hattie
squeezed my hand
before
she left the lunchroom.
Maybe it's not so obvious
me and my family
don't touch.
It's finally obvious to me:
Touching
feels good.

Testing It Out

"Pass the peas, please."
Mom hands me the bowl.
I grasp the edge
right by her hand.
My fingers close over hers.
"Sorry," she says,
and slips her hand
out from under mine.
"It's okay."

I serve myself some peas.
My hand is warm
where we touched.

Charts

Keeping
track
of medicines
takes
yellow
legal-size
paper.
Dates,
times,
and doses
are all
for pain.

I Pretend

If I get her to swallow the pills
at the exact right time
on every dose,
I'll cure her.
I pretend
I'm not pretending.

Hallucinations

Some days
the tiny pink pills
make Grandma Margie
pinch tiny bits of nothing
out of the air.
She pinches them between her finger and thumb,
then she eats them.
Pinching and eating.
"Don't, Grandma Margie," I beg.
But she nudges away my hand.
And keeps at it.
I see nothing
but Grandma Margie,

who's lost her mind
for the moment,
chewing on
the bits she's pinched.

Kinds

Of the bizillion kinds
of cancer,
Grandma Margie's type
is so rare
there isn't a cure.
Knowing this
special one
is in Grandma Margie
ends her chemotherapy
and sucks our last hope
out.

Explosion

"We just need
a different kind of treatment," says Gran Eula.
"No, I think we need
another opinion," says Mom.
"Why can't everyone
leave her alone," I yell to be heard.
"Because this is my daughter's life."
"Like you really think Kay doesn't
know that?" Mom runs to my defense.
"Don't you speak to me like that."
"When are you going to wake up and see
you
aren't in control?" asks Mom.
"And you are?"
"At least I'm not taking this out on a child."
"I'm not a child, Mom."
"So who's acting like a child
over not getting her way?" Gran Eula says.
Grandma Margie sits up
completely
on her own.
Silence.

We forgot she was there.
"I'll decide what to do about me."
Her voice shakes. "To your rooms."
Slam, slam, slam go our bedroom doors.
I am not a child.
Anymore.

A Day

A day goes by in silence
while Grandma Margie decides.
"No more treatments."
Gran Eula humphs.
"No more opinions."
Mom humphs.
"I just want my family
around me in peace."
Mom and Gran Eula
each raise an eyebrow.
That means truce.
"And young lady,
would you get me
some coffee?" Grandma Margie asks me.
"Certainly."

I head to the kitchen
with my nose in the air.

Mixing Her Coffee

The crystals dissolve.
No more medicine?
No more opinions?
But the cancer is still there.
I add the milk and sugar.
My lip trembles.
I am a child.

Sick of It

Gran Eula must have started it.
She doesn't touch Grandma Margie,
who rarely touches Mom,
who hardly ever touches me.
I'm sick of it.
We might not have
much time left
to touch.

I go straight to the top,
walk up behind
Gran Eula,
who's spooning bacon grease into the lard can,
and give her
a bear hug.
I'm surprised she's squishy at all.
She drops the spoon
and splatters fat across the counter.
I let go
and jump back.
My shaking hand
reaches for the counter
and misses.
Gran Eula turns around,
steps forward,
and hugs me close.

Skin and Bones

It seems
bones and skin
are all that are left.
My Grandma Margie

is a delicate pile
of bones,
which clatter
when we roll
her over
to air
her bedsores.

Air-conditioning

We keep the air down to sixty all the time now
for Grandma Margie.
A lot of times she's super hot.
Sometimes I get so cold
I have to sit on the burning sidewalk,
humidity pressing down tons,
until my whole body sweats.
Water dumps out of every pore
like all of me is crying,
while Grandma Margie is being preserved
in the air-conditioning.

Incomplete

Incomplete
assignments,
reports,
essays,
projects.
My report card
lists a row of
*Incomplete*s,
not the Fs I deserve,
just *incomplete*s
that I can make up
later.
I'm incomplete now.
What will I be later?

Missing Parts

"Here."
I give Hattie my rolled-up drawing.
"There's lots of organs
I haven't drawn yet."
I drag my tennis shoe

on the linoleum.
"No problem."
Hattie snaps the rubber band
squeezing the paper.
"I can finish it," she says,
"and we can put
both our names
on it.
I didn't have a good idea
for the science project.
This is a big help
to me."
"Did you know
Deb, Sheray, and David
are doing the other parts?"
"Yeah."
"But it's fine
for us to do this part together."
"Great." She shifts her books. "Well, see you."
Hattie walks down the hall
with my drawing.
I feel more empty
than my outline
on that piece of paper.
I realize

I never
drew in
my heart.

No More

She says,
"I don't want
any more visitors,"
which is good,
because no one
seems up
to visiting.

Today

This morning
Gran Eula patted Grandma Margie's shoulder,
and Grandma Margie hugged Mom.
"Love you," they each whispered
when I kissed them
on the cheek.

I headed off to school
almost happy.

Examples of Singular Verb Forms Ending in S

A family loveS.
A teacher careS.
A pastor prayS.
A cancer killS.
A God sayS.
A girl surviveS.
She hopeS.

Leaving

She's leaving.
I don't say anything
to anyone,
but I see it
when she looks past us
to something else.
She hurts so much,
she has to leave

for herself
and us.

Preparations

Her whole life
Gran Eula has asked Grandma Margie
questions.
Stuff like Mom has asked me.
> Would you like this lunch box or that one?
> Would you like braids today or barrettes?
> Would you like a slumber party
> or dinner out for your birthday?

But none of those
are like these questions.
> Would you like intervention or a living will?
> Would you like flowers or donations?
> Would you like cremation or burial?

Mom and I sit in my room until
Gran Eula is done asking
and Grandma Margie is done
answering.

"I could never ask her
about this stuff," says Mom.
"Me, either."
"Thank God
for Gran Eula, hon."

The Truth

When I think Grandma Margie's sleeping,
I whisper,
"I need you."
She whispers back with her eyes closed,
"I know.
I need you, too."
I slip my hand into hers.
We hold on
to what we have
for right now.

The Others

Grandma Margie sighs.
"You know

your grandpa and great-grandpa
are waiting for me?"
I nod and bite my lip.
Why can't we all be together now?
"We'll all be together in heaven
one day," she whispers.
"Me, too?" I squeak.
She doesn't answer.
She's asleep.

The Nurse

She comes to our house
to check on Grandma Margie,
check on us,
check Grandma Margie's pulse,
check our charts,
and give us a pamphlet
on recognizing death,
like we aren't already
seeing it.

Can't Make It

We hardly get to church
because we can't leave Grandma Margie.
I haven't been to Sunday School
since forever.
Someone took over teaching
for Mom weeks ago.
Miss Martha Faye
sent me a letter.
She said to call anytime.
But I don't feel close to her.
It's hard to imagine
beautiful Miss Martha Faye
has a clue
about how ugly
cancer is.

Missing Out

I'm missing school, too.
Mr. Hoeksema sends a card.
Everyone signed it:
"To: Kay, a real peach

From:
Deb,
Sheray,
Ms. Reynolds,
Mr. Arnold,
Mr. Ball,
David,
Ms. Certel,
Hattie,"
and everyone else.
"WE MISS YOU!"
it says really big.
That does it.
I sniffle,
then start crying.
Pretty soon
I'm bawling my head off
in my room.
I keep it up
until,
finally,
Mom comes in.
She doesn't say one word
but hugs me tightly
while I cry

for myself,
finally showing
I'm not fine.
I have to cry.
I'm not perfect.
I
need
her.
And
she
actually cries
too.

Part

Touching,
crying,
and needing
don't mean
you're not perfect.
They're part
of being
people.
Good parts.

School Conference

Mom takes time
to go in and meet
with my teachers.

I try to guess
all Grandma Margie's needs
before she says,
"Water,"
"A blanket,"
"Maybe a cracker."

Plus
I vacuum,
scrub the shower,
and wipe the mirror clean.

Ugh.
I frown at myself.
What are they
going to tell
Mom?

Okay

She sits down next to me
on the porch.
"Hon, it'll be okay."
I put my head on my knees.
"All your teachers
were very understanding."
I sweep a bull ant off my foot
and rub the sting.
"You can even work during
the summer if necessary."
"Okay." I stick and unstick
my sweaty knees.
"Just don't worry."
"I'm not," I say.
I hardly care.

Enough

"They did suggest
visiting the school counselor."
"I don't want to."
"I told them

you'd say that."
"How'd you know?"
"Well, you are my daughter, hon.
I told them
you have your family,
a few friends,
and our church and pastor.
That's probably enough.
Am I right?"
"Absolutely."

My Mother

"No more meds yet.
Her dose doesn't run out
for fifteen minutes," says the nurse.

My mom
grabs her white lapel
and hisses,
"Don't you give me that
crap.
Give it to my mother!
Now!"

The nurse gives it
right away.

Gurgle

When I wake,
I think
I hear
Gran Eula's coffeepot
gurgling.
But it's
Grandma Margie's
breath
trying
so hard
to
get
in
and
back
out.

Aside

Mom pulls me aside.
"If you want to be in
with Grandma Margie,
you have to be strong."
I nod.
"You can't make an upsetting scene."
I nod.
"You have to help
make this a peaceful, quiet time
for her."
I nod,
and she holds my hand
as we go into the living room.

Quietly

Grandma Margie
opens her watery eyes.
"It's time to go."

I want to beg,
"Don't go!"

But Mom and Gran Eula don't.
For her sake.
So I swallow those words down
and choke out,
"Good-bye, Grandma Margie."

She smiles at me,
reaches up,
and pats my cheek.

I lean down
and kiss hers.
Mom cradles Grandma Margie's head
and kisses her stubbly hair.
Gran Eula kisses her right hand
and holds it to her heart.

"I love you each," Grandma Margie whispers.
She takes a deep breath in,
and as she lets the air slowly out
she floats out of her body.
I can't see her doing it,
but I feel it.
Quietly
she floats to God.
Her left hand

rests
on my yellow scarf.

No!

She's gone.

"No!"
I stomp my feet.
"No, Grandma Margie.
Don't leave me.
Please don't.
Don't go!"
I cram my fingers
into my hair
and pull hard.
Harder.
The pain
isn't enough
to cover my heart pain.
Mom and Gran Eula
don't even look at me.
They are on the other side of the bed
sobbing

into each other's shoulders
I let go of my hair.
"Grandma Margie," I whimper,
and lay my head
on her empty spot
where her breast used to be.
"Please come back."
I weep.

Amazing

She wasn't scared.
She did the scariest thing
in the world,
dying,
and she wasn't scared
a
bit.

The Body

Mom pulls me up.
"She's gone, hon."
She tugs me close,
and we cry together.
Gran Eula joins us.
We make a tight circle
and hold each other up.
"Her pain,
her sadness,
and her cancer
are gone," says Gran Eula.

I look over at the body.
That isn't Grandma Margie.
It doesn't even
look like her
anymore.

I pull in a rattly breath.
It's just
an
empty
body.

Three

The three of us
on Earth.
Me, Mom, Gran Eula.

Completely miserable.

The three of them
in heaven.
Grandma Margie, Grandpa, and Great Grandpa.

Perfectly happy.

The Last Prayer

God,
take
good
care
of
my
Grandma
Margie.

Zip

Mom makes me go to my room
when the police and coroner come.
I sit on my shaking hands.
What if they think
we killed
Grandma Margie?

Mumble, mumble, mumble
seeps through my door.
Then one long *zip,*
and it's quiet.

I come out into the empty living room.
"No, no, no," I whisper
until I shove back the curtain.
Outside
it's black.
In the circle
of yellow porch light
Mom and Gran Eula are
holding hands.
They're not wearing handcuffs.

Beds

"Why don't you try to rest, Kay?"
Mom snivels and turns down my bed.
"I . . . I need a tissue first."
I stumble past
Gran Eula,
who's crying
while she
straightens and tucks the sheets
on Grandma Margie's
empty hospital bed.
She fluffs her pillow
and pats it.
A big sob sticks in my throat.
Gran Eula
is making up
her daughter's bed
for the last time.

Time Passing

Mom
by my bed.
Roll over.
Cry
into my pillow.
The phone
rings.
Gran Eula
by my bed.
A glass
of water.
Roll over.
Whispers.
Mom.
Gran Eula.
Me.
Crying.

Questions

Mom drives.
Gran Eula and I
sit in the back
and stare out the window.
What's happened
the last couple days
since Grandma Margie died?
I don't remember daytime
or night.
It's just one long moment
of crying and sleeping.
My eyelids
press to stay open
in my puffy face.
We pull into the funeral parlor.
Why do they call it that?
Funeral parlor.
How many parlors do they have?
How many dead people are here?
"Come on, Kay."
Mom holds my door open.
I get out
without a question.

Fake

Ffwwaaahh.
Gran Eula
opens the funeral parlor door.
It sounds like all the air
was sealed out
of the building
and it's trying to rush in.
We step into the dark hallway.
Fwooom.
The door shuts
behind us
automatically.
Mom speaks to the bald man
at the desk.
"Please follow me." He smiles
fake.
Down the dark hall,
into a room.
I peek around Mom and Gran Eula.
So this is a parlor, maybe.
Big curtains,
flowers.
Mom steps over to a pew and sits down.

My eyes jar to a stop.
Grandma Margie
is lying in a casket,
smiling
fake.

Disgusting

Gran Eula
whispers to Mom
in the pew.
I wander
over to the coffin.
I don't want to see,
but I have to.
The red wood is super shiny.
The white velvet inside is beautiful.
My eyes creep closer
to her face.
That is not
Grandma Margie!
It's not even
her dead body.
I make myself check again.

It is.
But whatever they've done to her
is
disgusting.
Thick blue eye shadow
and reddened cheeks.
Her skin
looks like
my finger
would stick in it
if I touched her.
And her lips are stretched
gross
into a smile that's like a wide grimace.
She's going to have that look
stuck
forever.
If this is what her outsides look like,
what did they do to her insides?
Like her heart?
Bile burns my throat.
"What did they do to you,
Grandma Margie?"

Yelling at Mom in the Ladies' Room

"I'm mad the bald man
came over to me and said,
'She's not suffering anymore,'
because I am.

"I'm mad some stupid mortician
made her smile
that stupid way.

"I'm mad she's not
in her body
anymore.

"I'm mad at God
for taking her
to himself.

"I'm mad
that
I'm mad."
Mom pulls me close.
"Me, too, hon."

Dead

Why do
the fresh flowers
smell
a little
bit dead?
Why does the
bald funeral director
look
a little
bit dead?
Why does the
organ
sound just like
death?
Isn't Grandma Margie's
being here dead
enough?

A Kiss

We stand
stiff
next to the open coffin.
Right where the director told us.
And the people start to come.

People from church.
Smile.
Hug.
Next.
Look in the coffin.

Her friends and neighbors.
Smile.
Hug.
Next.
Look in the coffin.

People I don't even know.
Smile.
Hug.
Next.
Look in the coffin.

Last in line,
Grandma Margie's old, old friend
Orpha.
Smile.
Hug.
Leans into the coffin
and gives Grandma Margie
a kiss
on the lips.

I run to the bathroom
and am sick
because I didn't have the guts
to even touch
Grandma Margie.

When I come back,
the coffin's closed.

I'm stuck.

Everyone is sitting down,
and our pastor
is walking up to the podium.
Everyone is staring
at me.

Pastor stops
and comes over.
He doesn't say anything.
He puts his arm
around my shoulder.
That blocks my view of everyone else.
He helps me to the pew
where my family's sitting.
He gives me a squeeze
before I sit down.
"There you go, Kay."
I look up at him.
"Thanks."
I really mean it.

The Service

Pastor speaks.
Gran Eula speaks.
Mom speaks.
But I hear
nothing
but myself.
Grandma Margie,

I
miss
you.

First

Gran Eula
looks so old
muttering,
"It should have been me first.
It should have been me."

What's it like
to bury your child?
Maybe
Gran Eula
should
have been first.

The Receiving Line

This
isn't for us.
We know
Grandma Margie's dead.
This
is for them,
the other people who knew
and loved her,
to know
she really is gone.
But the line
is so long.
Friend
after friend.
Their grief
tries
to join ours.
But it can't even
come close.
She was my grandma,
her mother,
and her daughter.

No one
can feel that.

They Came

Mr. Hoeksema
and Ms. Certel
wait,
last.
Finally
they get to me
and hold me
in a hug.
They came
here
for me.
"Oh, Kay," says Ms. Certel.
"We are so sorry," says Mr. Hoeksema.
"Thank you."
"Deb, Sheray, David,
and Hattie were here," says Ms. Certel.
"Really?"
"They send their love," Mr. Hoeksema says.

"David's mother drove them back to school
as soon as the service ended."
"That's nice."
"They couldn't wait."
Ms. Certel pats my shoulder.
"Right.
This is taking forever."
"We'll see you in class, Peach. Take care."
"Bye."

That's it.
Everyone has left
for the grave site
or they are waiting outside
to follow us there.
Everyone's gone
but Gran Eula,
Mom,
me,
and the casket.

The Hall Mirror

Black
Dress
High
Heels
Splotchy
Face
I hate
This place.

Mom

Mom
sits in the dark corner,
alone,
waiting for the director.
She's crying hard,
and it hits me
hard:
My mom's
mom
is dead,
but I

still
have
mine.
Maybe
she needs me.
I go
hug
her
and
hug
her.
She is
more perfect
than ever.
Exactly
how
I love her.

The Hearse

Another silent drive,
but this time
a row of cars is following us.
It stretches back

farther than I can see.
The black hearse is ahead of us.
I hate that ugly thing.
People slow down
in the lanes next to us
and gawk.
It's hard not to make faces
at them.
Gran Eula
reaches over
and squeezes my hand.
"It's okay for them to look, Kay.
People need to see death."
I squeeze her hand back.
Well, I'm not going to look at them.
We turn into the graveyard
and weave through the little streets
packed with tombstones.
Mom stops
next to a black canopy.
We're here.

The Burial

My fake smile
covers my heart
like the green plastic grass
covers the hole
no one wants to see.

Herein

Herein lies
a daughter,
a mother,
a grandmother,
a part of me.

Later

"They'll lower the casket later," says Gran Eula.
"They will," says Mom.
But why should I trust
two guys with shovels
who smoked, whispered, and chuckled

the whole time
our pastor was praying?

The Gathering

I want everyone to leave our house.
I don't want them saying,
"She was a lovely woman."
I don't want them dropping bean dip
off their chips
onto her chair.
"Have some of Barbara's chicken casserole."
"No," I say.
The mushy chicken smell
mixes with their perfume
and bad breath.
My stomach lurches.
"Get out!" I shout.
Mom hurries me to my room.
"I'll stay with her," says Gran Eula.
Mom goes back to the guests,
while Gran Eula tucks me into bed
like a baby.
Then she draws the blinds

and turns off the lights.
"No harm done, sugarplum," she whispers
as I fall asleep.

How Dare They?

First thing I see
when I go to the bathroom
in the middle of the night
is three toothbrushes.
Grandma Margie's is in the trash can,
lying on top of garbage.
I pick it up
and slam it into our holder
right next to mine.

Crunch

I stop in the kitchen
to get a drink of water,
and there he is.
That giant cockroach
is sitting in the middle

of our floor.
He's at least two inches.
His antennae shift.
His back end hikes up.
Then he actually takes off.
Flies right at me.
I'm batting the air
with a pot holder,
I'm so ticked.
He lands back on the floor
and
I stomp him
as hard as I can.
He crunches under my slipper.
I killed him good for Grandma Margie.
I scrape the bottom of my slipper
against the lip of the garbage can,
get a sip of water,
and go back to bed.

Losing My Mind

This morning
they find me
on her bed,
not crying
but breathing,
smelling her pillow,
and filling myself
with Grandma Margie's scent.

Tonight
they get me up
because I won't
and can't
on my own.
They put me
in my bed
and wash her pillow.

Afterward

We are walking
through the house,
barely eating,
whenever and whatever,
sitting,
thinking,
no words,
just tears.
And if we happen
to bump into each other,
we hug.

A Card

I get one card
that says,
"I'm sorry for your loss.
My mom died from it too.
Hattie."

No Wonder

No wonder
she dresses differently.
She doesn't have a mom.
No wonder
her period started without her realizing it.
She doesn't have a mom.
No wonder she's so quiet.
She's missing her mom.
No wonder
she floats.

Fishing

I make it to the canal
with my rod
but forget the bread.

I lower the empty hook
into the water
for no reason
except it's what we always did.
The fish gulp

at the nothingness.
Until one catches
its open mouth
on the hook

I pull the fish in,
unhook it,
and watch it breathe,
straining to breathe,
in my hands.

I throw it back
into the canal
and watch it
swim away.

The Newspaper

In the coffin,
in the earth,
is my Grandma Margie.
Not because "she lost her fight,"
but because it was time.
The hand
of God

said it was best,
and that's what she'd tell
the newspaper.

Shoes

"They're worn out," says Gran Eula.
"They're not the right size," says Mom.

"Like I care they have holes?
Like I care they don't fit?
Like, would you listen to me
and just try to get it!"

I stomp away from them
in Grandma Margie's shoes.

Wobbling

I cross my legs
up onto my blow-up chair.
Her shoes are safe
on me.
"Hon?" Mom pushes open my door.

"Yeah."
"I get it."
"Good."
I rock my chair
like Grandma Margie did
that one time.
I wobble it around,
and my anger wobbles away.
I smile.
"What are you doing?" Mom asks.
"Remembering."
She reaches for my hand.
"Tell me about it, Kay."

Deb Calls

"Sorry I didn't get to say hi
at the funeral, Kay.
Sorry about your Grandma Margie."
"Thanks."
"Sorry I haven't called."
"It's okay."
"I didn't really know what to say."
"Me, either."

"I wanted to say
I know your grandma
did everything she could,
because she loved you,
and that was really brave."
"Thanks, Deb."
"And I wanted to tell you
I broke up with David."
"Oh."
"But he's still working on the science project
with me, Sheray, and Hattie."
"Great," I say.
"He told me to say he says 'Hi.'"
"You can say 'Hey' back for me."
"Okay."
Silence.
"She's pretty nice," says Deb,
"Hattie, I mean.
Once you get to know her."
"I know."
"I told her sorry about the crawdad,
and she said it was no big deal
right away."
"Cool."
"Well, see you in school."

"Yeah," I say.
"Thanks for calling."

Giving to Charity

Gran Eula
is packing up Grandma Margie's things.
"Have to get our ducks in a row."

When she isn't looking,
I nab Grandma Margie's glasses,
her sweater,
the photo of us fishing,
her bandanna,
and the yellow scarf I knitted for her.

I squirrel them away
into the very back of my
underwear drawer.

When I reach past Gran Eula's back
to snatch Grandma Margie's brush,
she grabs my wrist.
"I don't want it to go to charity," I beg.

"I want it," she says,
and I don't argue.

My Pastor

He preaches
God's sovereignty
and Christ's redemption.
He preaches,
and I pray to believe
all the goodness
of it
so I'm ready to die
like Grandma Margie was.

Working

Mom clicks
at her computer.
She's only taken
a couple days off.
Clickety, clickety, clickety.
"Thanks for always

working so hard," I say.
"Sometimes
it's just easier
to keep working," she says.
"I get it."

Knit Together

Needles
plunged into a ball.
Loops of love
left in Grandma Margie's basket,
a soft, unfinished blue angora blanket.
The stitches
are so even and beautiful.
She buried
her ends
as she finished each skein.
So all the loose threads
are safe,
deep inside
where they can't unravel.
Mom and Gran Eula
can't even touch the blanket,

but I will try
not to drop
a stitch.

Her Favorite

One
silver can of baby peas.
I'm bawling in the grocery aisle
while I hold
one
silver can of baby peas.

Sweetness

Grandma Margie left her sweetness
with us.
It's in Gran Eula
when she strokes my head.
It's in Mom
when she says I look beautiful today,
and it's in me

when I can tell them both,
"I love you."

Sunshower

I smell it.
The golden sweet air
rushes by,
bulging full.
I breathe in
and feed the deepest spots of my lungs.
The rain sprinkles
while the sun shines
even more brilliantly
through the water droplets.
I stand on the sidewalk
in front of our house
looking up into the sunshower.
It pats my face
like Grandma Margie's hand
on my cheek.

Best

No more pain for her.
No more tears for her.
No more death
ahead of her.

We are touching.
We are saying
we love each other.

This is all I can see
about it being best.
Maybe someday
I'll figure out more.
But for now
I think I've been given
the grace of faith.

Radar

Somehow
we all end up in the living room
at the same time.
Mom turns the TV on.

M★A★S★H.
Gran Eula is the first to smile.
"My daughter loved Radar."
Mom is the first to laugh.
"My mother did love Radar."
Grandma Margie would have laughed.
It's okay.
I bust up laughing on my beanbag chair.
Grandma Margie
really
loved Radar.

Telling the Truth

I open my eyes.
Mom is standing over me
smiling.
"What?" I whisper.
She sits on the edge of my bed.
"You are really wonderful," she says.
"I was lying in bed thinking it,
and I had to come tell you."
Her fingers
weave through
my hair on my pillow.

"I love you
so much, Kay."
"I love you, too, Mom."
I pull the covers up
over my mouth and say,
"And I think you're perfect."
"What?"
"I do." I reach out and hold her hand.
"Honey, I'm so far from perfect.
One day you'll see."
"I don't think so."
"You will. And I hope then
you'll still love me."
"Always, Mom."
Always.

2:00 A.M.

I dream she's alive,
but wake and see
she really isn't at my door.

I curl up
in her chair.

The arms hug me close.
The blank TV screen
shows
my reflection
is a tiny bit like
my Grandma Margie's.
Especially
my eyes.

Back to School

Going back to school means:
Mr. Ball's air freshener,
Ms. Certel's diet,
and Mr. Hoeksema calling me Peach.
But the important thing
happens on the bus.
I tell David,
"Sorry, this seat's saved
for Hattie."
He says,
"Cool," winks at me,
and walks on by.
How can he

still
be
so
cute?

First Sip

The waitress
in the noisy diner
brings us instant coffee by mistake.
Gran Eula and Mom don't look
at the cup.
So I tear the packet open,
clink the spoon,
and spin the coffee in circles.
I button Grandma Margie's sweater
up to my neck
and finger the knot
where I tied off the loose thread.
I fixed it best I could.
My first sip of coffee
is warm and sweet.

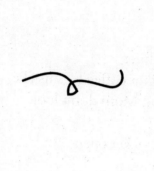

I loved growing up with my grandparents and great-grandparents living near our home in Miami. My house was far from school, so my family was my social life. Four generations headed to the beach, had picnics, and enjoyed the holidays together.

When I was fourteen, my maternal grandmother discovered a pea-size lump in her breast. It was sickening to imagine a surgeon cutting off part of her body. But that's what quickly happened. I spent a lot of time worrying whether I would get cancer one day. I wondered how this horrible thing could happen and why it did. The huge scar, the radiation marks, and my grandmother's reaction to chemo were ugly and overwhelming.

With remission, normal life resumed. However, the cancer recurred five years later. I was living with my grandparents to attend the nearby university. I watched my grandmother's body decline and her faith remain firm. She seemed to grow smaller and weaker, while the cancer grew bigger and stronger. Her life was exhausted. She died in peace with family around her. At the funeral I angrily asked her pastor why God had taken her. He told me I already knew why. I did, but it was hard to believe at that moment. I wanted my grandmother back.

Writing *Loose Threads* meant revisiting the joy and pain my family experienced together. The act of writing and the passage of time have helped me to appreciate, even more, the truths that give meaning to my life.

For more information about breast cancer and aring for a loved one with cancer, consult the fol-
owing resources.

Organization Web Sites

erican Cancer Society
p://www.cancer.org
800-ACS-2345
iformation concerning:
3reast Cancer Network
Site offers:
Breast Cancer Early Detection Shower Card
Breast Cancer Early Detection Bookmark

breastcancer.org
http://www.ibreast.org

Digital Breast Clinic
http://www.digitalclinic.com
713-383-7398

National Alliance of Breast Cancer Organizations
(NABCO)
http://www.nabco.org
1-800-719-9154

National Breast Cancer Awareness Month (NBCAM)
http://www.nbcam.org
Information concerning:
National Mammography Day

National Breast Cancer Coalition (NBCC)
http://www.natlbcc.org/homeindx.asp
202-296-7477

National Cancer Institute
http://www.nci.nih.gov
1-800-4-CANCER

National Coalition for Cancer Survivorship
http://www.cansearch.org
1-888-650-9127

Susan G. Komen Breast Cancer Foundation
http://www.komen.org
1-800-IM-AWARE
Information concerning:
Race for the Cure
Site offers:
Breast Self-exam Shower Card

Y-Me National Breast Cancer Organization
http://www.y-me.org
1-800-221-2141

Young Survival Coalition (YSC)
http://www.youngsurvival.org

Books and Pamphlets

Caregiving: A Step-by-Step Resource for Caring for the Person with Cancer at Home, by Peter S. Houts and Julia A. Bucher (American Cancer Society, 2001).

The Comfort of Home: An Illustrated Step-by-Step Guide for Caregivers, by Maria M. Meyer, with Paula Derr (Care Trust Publications, 1998).

Dr. Susan Love's Breast Book, 3rd revised edition, by Susan M. Love and Karen Lindsey (Perseus Book Group, 2000).

Share the Care: How to Organize a Group for Someone Who Is Seriously Ill, by Cappy Capossela and Sheila Warnock (Simon & Schuster, 1995).

"What About Me?" Booklet for Teenage Children of Cancer Patients, by Linda Leopold Strauss (Cancer Family Care, 1986), 513-731-3346.

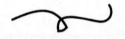